T0015286

# Download your free workout app!

**Step 1:** Remove the scratch layer below for your unique code:

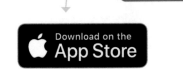
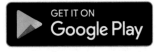

**Step 2:** Go to www.thewonderweeks .com/bty and register your book.

**Step 3:** Download the **Wonder Weeks - Back To You** App and follow the instructions.

**Step 4:** Click the "I have the book" button.

**Step 5:** Enter your email address and password you created when registering.

**Step 2:** Download the **Wonder Weeks - Back To You** App and follow the instructions.

**Step 3:** Click the "I have the book" button.

**Step 4:** Enter your unique code and email address.

**Step 5:** Verify your email address.

Now you have access to all the **Back To You** workouts. Enjoy the program!

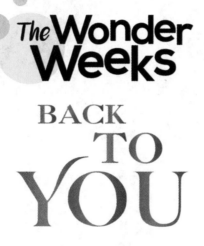

# BACK TO YOU

*ALSO AVAILABLE FROM THE WONDER WEEKS*

The Wonder Weeks: A Stress-Free Guide to Your Baby's Behavior

# The Wonder Weeks

# BACK TO YOU

## The Ultimate Recovery Program After Pregnancy

## XAVIERA PLOOIJ
### AND LAURENS MISCHNER

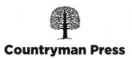

**Countryman Press**

*An Imprint of W. W. Norton & Company*
*Independent Publishers Since 1923*

For information about permission to reproduce selections from this book,
write to Permissions, Countryman Press, 500 Fifth Avenue, New York, NY 10110

For information about special discounts for bulk purchases, please contact
W. W. Norton Special Sales at specialsales@wwnorton.com or 800-233-4830

Countryman Press
www.countrymanpress.com

An imprint of W. W. Norton & Company, Inc.
500 Fifth Avenue, New York, NY 10110
www.wwnorton.com

978-1-68268-671-3

10 9 8 7 6 5 4 3 2 1

To our wonderful children—Thomas, Victoria, Sarah, Jack, and Floris—who will always live in our hearts

# CONTENTS

11 NOTE TO THE READER
12 FOREWORD

## 16 You and Your Brain
17 Come to Grips with Your Mom Brain: Put Your Mind at Ease
17 *The Wonder Weeks* Leap That Your Mom Brain Makes
19 Emotions Resulting from Your Mom Brain

## 21 You and Your Powerhouse
23 Your Powerhouse Explained
26 Pelvic Floor Muscles
26 The Pelvic Floor and Pregnancy
28 Rediscover the Connection Between the Pelvic Floor and Brain
30 The Pelvic Floor and Abdominal Muscles and the Pressure during Pregnancy
39 Everything Is Connected: The Domino Effect

## 40 You and Your Vagina
41 Your Vagina: No Pain and No Discomfort
50 10 Benefits of Sex for Women

## 51 You and Your Hormones
52 What Are Hormones?
53 These Hormones Play a Role after Childbirth
56 From a Major Increase during Pregnancy to a Drastic Drop after the Delivery

## 60 You and Your Mind
61 Back to You or a New You?
61 The Changes in You
65 From (Normal) Stress to Depression

## 71 The XL Fundamentals
72 The XL Fundamentals: For a Real Impact on You
73 That Means a Lot of Changes . . . Nope. It Doesn't.

## 74 XL Fundamental: Nutrition
75 10 Golden Nutrition Tips

**86  XL Fundamental: Rest and Relaxation**

87  Sleep

90  Relaxation

**93  XL Fundamental: Posture and Breathing**

94  Posture

104  Breathing

**108  XL Fundamental: Exercise and Training**

109  Exercise

111  Training

115  10 Golden Training Tips

**118  Let's Get Started: Your BTY Program**

121  The First Training Session of a New Block

124  Just Gave Birth or Gave Birth Years Ago

125  The Training Sessions after Your Self-Test

125  Your Results (After a Couple of Weeks)

126  When Are You Recovered?

**127  Activating, Loosening, and Demanding Functionality of the Muscles**

128  If Your Muscle Function Is Restricted

129  Activating and Loosening Do Wonders for Your Muscles

131  Activating Your Muscles: This Is How You Do It

131  Loosening Your Muscles: This Is How You Do It

133  Stretching: This Is How You Do It

134  Demanding Functionality: This Is How You Do It

**136  Your Daily Pelvic Floor Exercises**

137  How the Training Program Builds Your Pelvic Floor Muscles

139  Daily BTY Kegel Exercises

**145  The Correct Basic Training Posture**

146  Neutral Position

147  Imprint Position

148 Phase 1: Back

150 Postpartum Health Issues
152 Lacerations, Incisions, and Care
153 "Back" Tips from the Experts
156 Training in the "Back" Phase

170 Phase 2: To

171 Back to Work
172 Contraception after Childbirth
173 "To" Tips from the Experts
180 Training in the "To" Phase

218 Phase 3: You

219 Losing Weight . . . Bye-Bye, Pounds
221 "You" Tips from the Experts
222 Training in the "You" Phase

258 Test Yourself

259 Test: Stressful Life Events
260 Test: Are Your Pelvic Floor Muscles Strong Enough?
261 Test: How Big Is Your Diastasis Recti and How Strong is Your Linea Alba?
264 Test: Are you Suffering with a Prolapse (Sagging)?
265 Test: How Do You Breathe?
265 Test: Do You Breathe Optimally?
265 Back Mobility: Cat to Cow

267 Exercises

291 Before and After

295 AFTERWORD
296 ACKNOWLEDGMENTS
298 BIBLIOGRAPHY
301 INDEX

# NOTE TO THE READER

**B**ACK TO YOU is a general information resource about postpartum recovery; it is not a substitute for individual medical diagnosis or treatment. Each childbirth is different and each woman's recovery from childbirth is different. Neither the authors, nor the publisher, nor anyone else involved in the development, production, marketing, or distribution of this book can predict your postpartum experience or guarantee the results of following this program.

Check with your healthcare provider before you embark on any post-childbirth exercise program, and read any warning listed with any exercise in this book before you start that exercise. Some exercises are strongly discouraged for women with particular postpartum conditions, and even stretching can cause injuries if done incorrectly, especially when you are recovering from childbirth and if you have had a cesarean section. Consult your healthcare provider before resuming contraception and before ingesting or changing your diet to include significant amounts of any new food, any herbal or other supplement, or any other substance, especially if you are diabetic or suffer from an autoimmune or other health condition, if you are taking any prescription medication, if you are nursing, or if you have food or other allergies. **If you feel severely depressed or you have any doubt or concern about your own physical or emotional health or well-being during the postpartum period,** consult your healthcare professional. Do not hesitate to seek emergency care for your yourself if you think it may be needed.

As of press time, the URLs displayed in this book link or refer to existing websites. The publisher is not responsible for, and should not be deemed to endorse or recommend, any website other than its own or any other content available on the Internet or elsewhere, including, without limitation, any app, blog page, or information page that is not created by W. W. Norton. The authors also are not responsible for any material that they did not create.

# FOREWORD

## Facts

- Your body, mind, and even the structure of your brain change after childbirth.
- It takes months for your body to adjust to the new hormone levels.
- Pelvic floor muscles that don't recover can cause health conditions for life, including pain, bowel movement issues, fewer (or less intense) orgasms, and incontinence at a later age.
- Relationships change.
- The secure attachment with your baby can be affected if you don't recover properly.

Nine months on, nine months off. It is a well-known expression, but after your final checkup roughly six weeks after the birth, you are on your own. Postpartum recovery is just as complex for your mind and body as being pregnant is. And yet . . . you are left to figure it out by yourself. How can we leave women high and dry like that?

## THIS. MUST. CHANGE. THIS. WILL. CHANGE. NOW.

The Back To You program is revolutionary, and it will guide you to full recovery and even to a better version of yourself, both mentally as well as physically. Recovering after childbirth will be the new norm. You, your body, and any relationship you have deserve that. You have brought a miracle into the world, and now you deserve some support to get . . . Back To You.

You are holding a revolutionary program in your hands. Every mother knows that it's not only the position of your abdominal muscles that changes when you have a baby. It was like looking for hidden treasure, but with the best global experts, we have created Back To You. BTY looks at all sides of recovery and not only at reducing your dress size and getting a flat tummy. The superficial quick-fix programs that currently exist are a genuine insult to women who really want to recover. It takes a lot more to fully bounce back.

It was clearly obvious that we needed a BTY movement. All the experts we spoke to were almost begging for a program like this. It could really change the way women across the world recover. The first thing we heard from Sonia Bahlani, a highly distinguished gynecologist from New York, was: "Never before has there been a program that will be so beneficial to women. I feel honored that I can contribute to your book." And there were more comments like that:

"Finally, someone is talking about this."

"It's about time that this happened."

"This movement will be an amazing help to women across the globe."

There was no lack of encouragement. All these types of comments from these experts gave us the strength to keep going and develop this revolutionary program.

## BTY . . . Everything Is Connected

There was one thing that kept coming up during our discussions with the experts: The future of health is in thinking beyond boundaries. That is abundantly clear with recovery after pregnancy. Physicians need to look beyond their own specialty to see a person as a whole and how everything, and we mean everything, is connected and influences everything else. BTY, therefore, has been written based on that premise. Poor foot positioning can cause pelvic floor issues (pain during sex, difficulties with bowel movements). Stress about doing things wrong can cause pain in your thumbs. Sleepless nights can have such an effect on your hormones that it takes you longer to recover. Your maternal feelings can take over to such a degree that you forget yourself and your relationship. Your brain can suddenly perceive a different type, or other level, of empathy, whereby you could start doubting yourself beyond belief. Your nutrition can influence postpartum depression.

In short, everything is connected, both mentally as well as physically: there is no separating these two and all other associated factors if you want to understand the full picture.

## BTY . . . for XL Impact

We have developed the XL Fundamentals: the four factors that, individually, can have a massive impact on your recovery and health. But if you tackle them all at the same time, they can do wonders for your body and mind.

# BTY Is . . . Insight and Reassurance

BTY gives you:

1. Insight into the changes that have occurred in your brain, power-house (the muscles in your belly, back, midriff, and pelvis), vagina, hormone levels, and mind.

2. A complete program ranging from your pelvic floor muscles to your powerhouse to your mind. They will all be given a workout so that they become healthier and stronger.

## HOW TO USE YOUR BTY PROGRAM

DOWNLOAD THE FREE APP!

The BTY program consists of two parts: this book and the free training app. Download the app and use the unique code in the front of this book. You get this app for free from us because some things are simply easier to see than read about.

# The Back To You Program Consists of Three Phases

**BACK (0–6 WEEKS)** You take a little step back. Right now, it's about getting rest and making a connection: a connection with your baby and a connection with your new role as a mother. The exercises focus on the connection between your mind and your powerhouse.

**TO (7–24 WEEKS)** You gradually pick up your "normal" life again. You go back to work, to your social life, to yourself. The physical exercises work toward your stability and mobility. With the nonworkout, we work on your inner you and help you get back to the "normal" world in the process.

**YOU (25–40 WEEKS)** You are increasingly becoming your "new you" and finding your own strength. The exercises work intensively on that new you so that you will be healthier, stronger (both mentally as well as physically), and in better shape. You will become your new YOU! Or perhaps even a better version of yourself than ever before.

# The Basic Principles of the BTY Program

BTY has three basic principles for a good recovery. And here's the best bit: these three key points apply to your body as well as your mind, and we give them both a workout on all three points.

1. Connection
2. Pressure distribution
3. Full range of motion (from relaxing completely to tightening completely)

# YOU AND YOUR BRAIN

We all know that your uterus becomes a whole lot bigger during pregnancy, your feet can get a size bigger, your skin stretches, you could get permanent stretch marks, and your hormones change. What lots of people don't realize, however . . . drum roll . . . is that your brain also changes before and after childbirth! It really does. The structure and composition of the brain alters in a way that can only happen to women when they have been pregnant and have given birth to a child. Wow. The brain changes for a reason. It makes you more empathic, more alert, sharper, and makes you rearrange your priorities somewhat as compared to before. All this happens so that you can make the best start as a mother. But all those changes, the new brain skills, can take some getting used to!

## Come to Grips with Your Mom Brain: Put Your Mind at Ease

We still actually know very little about the way pregnancy affects the brain. In fact, the first studies are only a few years old, and that's why you don't hear much about them. Many physicians and practitioners are unaware of these studies or believe that the information should only be shared once we can answer all the questions. That's all well and good, but on the other hand, it could take decades for us to completely understand the mom brain. In the meantime, moms are left with certain questions and emotions, while an understanding of the maternal brain could make all the difference. In any case, know that you are not the issue, you are not emotionally unstable, nor is it a form of "doubteritis." However crazy it sounds, what you are feeling now makes you a better mother and is natural, biological process. Almost all moms have these feelings simply because that's how the brain is now programmed. In *Back To You*, we describe what's currently known about the mom brain and, even more important, what you can do to gain a permanent grip on your new mom brain. You should be reassured when you understand the changes in your brain. You are not the issue; it is purely a biological and chemical change in your brain.

## *The Wonder Weeks* Leap That Your Mom Brain Makes

*The Wonder Weeks* tells you all about the leaps your baby makes. Or should we say, the 10 timed brain changes your baby goes through. You'll first notice your baby is upset and exhibiting the three Cs: Crying, Clinginess, and

# SCIENTIFIC RESEARCH ON THE MOM BRAIN

Until fairly recently, scientists have given little attention to the effects of pregnancy on the brain. Most of the research was carried out by men, and there wasn't much focus on the woman herself. The research that has been done solely looked at the belly containing the growing baby. That seems logical, really, but it's also the reason that we don't know much about postpartum recovery. In 2016, the first really significant research into the mom brain was conducted by Dr. Elseline Hoekzema, a neuroscientist from Leiden University (the Netherlands). She was the first to discover that there are significant changes in the maternal brain after childbirth, and these can last for at least two years or even be permanent. These changes play a crucial role in the transition from woman to mother.

The brain consists of gray and white matter. The gray matter consists of neuronal cell bodies, and the white matter consists of long fibers, which are extensions of the nerve cells. After childbirth, there is a notable difference in the gray matter in the part responsible for social cognition, or empathy, the way you understand how others are feeling. That change in gray matter may not seem logical at first because the gray matter diminishes in that specific area. It decreases, but you could say it also improves and gets sharper. It seems this reduction in gray matter can cause the brain to become specialized. This allows women to better adapt to motherhood and better respond to their baby's needs. The development of the mom brain really is remarkable!

The difference in the brain scans of women who have never been pregnant was so clear that a computer algorithm could see by the brain whether someone had ever been pregnant and given birth. That might not be that surprising, actually. The hormonal changes during pregnancy are so strong that they can only be compared to those of puberty. And even after puberty you see a reorganization, a restructuring of the brain because of that peak in hormones. If you look at it from an evolutionary perspective, you could say that as a mother you will face different kinds of challenges, have to deal with problems differently, and will set other priorities. Your altered brain composition, your mom brain, makes that possible.

Crankiness. It makes perfect sense, really, considering the brain changes mean your baby experiences the world differently (a new perceptual ability), and that is scary for your child. Once your baby has gotten used to the new experiences, you will notice they can suddenly do all kinds of new things (new skills) they couldn't do before the brain change.

Let's look at your mom brain. It undergoes changes, which means you perceive the world differently. This can be scary, and it is often expressed through Crying, becoming a little listless (Clinginess), and mood changes (Crankiness). As a mom, you are actually taking a leap, too! It's not the same leap your baby goes through, of course, but it is comparable. *The Wonder Weeks* does not tell you how to reduce the bouts of crying or give you a miracle cure to finally get your baby to sleep. *The Wonder Weeks* offers parents across the world an insight into the changes in the brain, which enables parents to understand what's going on and be less insecure in their role as parents. This shows that simply understanding a complex biological process can be enough to provide support and alleviate doubts. The same applies to you and your mom brain!

# Emotions Resulting from Your Mom Brain

Great, now you have a better understanding of what other people mean, you are more aware of certain emotional signals, and you are more empathic. You have been transformed into a superwoman. And yet, you might not always experience it that way. That is perfectly normal and part of being a mom. Except for a few women who have total confidence in themselves and who don't experience a dark cloud moment, every new mother doubts herself, her family, or even her baby at times. It's a completely taboo subject, but that's the harsh reality. Almost everyone doubts themselves at some point. Almost everyone worries they'll not be good enough at the massive task of raising a child. At some point, almost every woman thinks it might not have been such a great idea to have had children. Have you ever heard about this? Probably not. We don't like discussing these feelings. And that's a shame because they are part of having a child, too. The major downside of not talking about these feelings of self-doubt is that it only makes them worse. Almost everyone has doubts, is insecure, and has very difficult times. And now we know that we can place part of the blame on the mom brain, this biological process should reassure you. You are not the issue; your brain has simply changed.

## YOUR BRAIN OR YOUR MIND?

Hmm . . . once again you see how everything in our body is connected. Your brain is subject to changes, and that can have a significant impact on how you feel, your approach to life, your emotions, and all other aspects of "you" that we can't pin on a body part. You can read more about all the changes that commonly play a big role when you have become a mother in "You and Your Mind" on page 60.

# YOU AND YOUR POWERHOUSE

Let's be honest, bringing a child into the world is like an Olympic sport. And an Olympic sport can be hard on your body. You will see most of the effects of the pregnancy on your belly. That makes perfect sense considering your uterus is inside your belly and where you carried your baby for nine months. Your uterus grew a whole lot during pregnancy, which put a massive amount of pressure on your pelvis and pelvic floor.

And let's clear up a myth and send it to the world of fallacies where it belongs: a pregnancy does not only affect your pelvis, even if that's generally the main focus. Your pelvis (pelvic floor) is directly connected to your abdominal muscles, your back muscles, and your midriff (diaphragm). You can't consider these four parts as isolated elements if you want a full and healthy recovery after your pregnancy. They work together, reinforce each other, and if one is weak, the others pay the price.

These four parts all form your powerhouse. Your powerhouse influences, and is influenced by, all your other body parts. Everything is connected, and everything affects everything else.

The Olympic feat you have just performed will have an impact on your body for a long time after the birth. In fact, without training you could experience lifelong consequences of your pregnancy, which is not the case when you make a conscious effort to recover. "Accept it because that's just how it is" is, therefore, myth number two.

Many of the effects (diastasis recti, hernia, or a prolapse; see pages 30–37) that you could suffer from for the rest of your life are the result of the struggle between the internal pressure and the strength of your powerhouse. When your powerhouse faces pressure from the inside, it must be strong enough to cope with that pressure. It is a misconception that the internal pressure goes away after the pregnancy. We experience this type of internal pressure every day; for example, when we sneeze, burst into laughter, or jump. These are the types of situations when it is imperative for your powerhouse to be functioning at its best so that you don't leak any urine when you sneeze, laugh, or jump.

Your powerhouse consists of:
- Your diaphragm (your midriff)
- Your abdominal muscles
- Your back muscles
- Your pelvis (pelvic floor)

You could see these four parts together as a house, in a way. Your diaphragm is at the top, which you could see as your powerhouse's roof. The foundation,

## Your Powerhouse

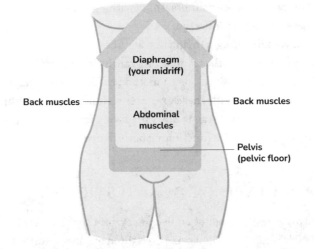

the underside of your house, is formed by your pelvis (pelvic floor). You could compare the walls at the front to your vertical abdominal muscles, the walls at the back to your back muscles, and the side walls to your oblique abdominal muscles. A powerhouse is only a powerhouse when all the parts are doing their job. It's no good having sturdy foundations with good walls but a leaking roof. If your walls aren't any good, how will you support your roof? And if your walls and roof are fine but standing on a sinking foundation, your house is useless.

# Your Powerhouse Explained

### 1. Your Diaphragm—The Roof of Your Powerhouse

Your diaphragm (midriff) is at the top of your powerhouse. It is a dome-shaped muscle, a type of partition between your lungs and your abdominal cavity that allows your lungs to expand and shrink. Each time you inhale, your lungs fill up with air, increasing the content and with that the size of the chest cavity at the expense of the contents of your abdominal cavity. With each inhalation the pressure on your powerhouse increases, and the pressure decreases each time you exhale. This is an extremely healthy and natural process.

You can feel the relationship between your diaphragm and your pelvic floor. Each time you inhale (mainly with abdominal breathing), your pelvic floor moves downward slightly, and each time you exhale, it rises somewhat. Inhaling and exhaling cause an exchange of pressure in your abdominal cavity, and that's how it should be.

You can influence your diaphragm through good breathing practices (see page 104).

And you can influence your breathing with a good straight posture. *Once again . . .* everything is connected.

To allow your diaphragm to function at its best and work together with the rest of your powerhouse, the training program includes posture and breathing exercises, and we have developed a method to loosen your diaphragm (see below). You can start with these exercises right after childbirth; they will relax you and are a great way to start preparing for the real training to get that taut, lovely, and fully functioning powerhouse.

## YOUR DIAPHRAGM AND STRESS

If you are stressed, your shoulders, neck, and jaw could become cramped. Your diaphragm can also tighten when you suffer from stress! Loosening your diaphragm gives an instant feeling of calm and relaxation. You can do this by placing four fingers just under your rib cage and pushing your fingers inward slightly. Then using your fingers, rub back and forth along your ribs.

## 2. Your Abdominal Muscles—The Side Walls and Front Facade of Your Powerhouse

It makes perfect sense that your abdominal muscles had a tough time during the pregnancy. Their relative positions changed. The vertical muscles are normally reasonably close to the surface in neat rows, but they were forced apart as the uterus grew.

Your oblique abdominal muscles are underneath the vertical abdominal muscles. Of all your abdominal muscles, these had the least direct "trouble" from the pregnancy. And yet they are often unable to do what they did before the pregnancy and have become weaker. You use your oblique abdominal muscles when you make a turning motion. Your ever-growing womb restricted that turning motion, which means you probably did it less during pregnancy.

The transverse abdominal muscle is the deepest layer of abdominals, running like a thick belt around your belly, and it was stretched a whole lot during the pregnancy. And that is precisely the abdominal muscle that is largely responsible for your stability and a flat-looking stomach.

When you start the training program, you will notice there are several abdominal muscle exercises. Each exercise tackles a specific abdominal muscle. You will also use your abdominal muscles with all the turning, or rotating, movements we ask you to do. People used to believe that you shouldn't make any rotating movements just after having a baby because that puts pressure on the vertical abdominal muscles. That view has changed. You can't escape the fact that you make rotating movements in daily life.

### 3. Your Back Muscles—The Rear Facade of Your Powerhouse

Your back had a lot to cope with during your pregnancy, too. Your uterus is connected to your lower back with round ligaments, and all that weight "hanging" at the front of your body pulled your back forward. That is why you often see women in the typical pregnancy posture: hollow lower back and belly forward. You should avoid standing like that during your entire pregnancy, but that's easier said than done. Your long muscles in your lower back start at the bottom by your pelvis and run along your spine. During pregnancy, the weight pulls the pelvis forward, and if you don't pay attention to your posture, you will automatically slouch, or hollow, your back. As a result, almost every woman's back muscle shortens in the final months of pregnancy. It is tight and needs to regain its former length through the right exercises and correct body posture.

### 4. Your Pelvis (Pelvic Floor)—The Foundation of Your Powerhouse

Your pelvis forms the base of your powerhouse. Your pelvis contains your uterus, where your baby grew for nine months, and it got a whole lot heavier. That resulted in shifts in the pressure on the pelvis. Think about it: when you are not pregnant, your uterus is so small, it sits under your pubic bone; and by the end of your pregnancy, your uterus is so big that it almost reaches your midriff. Your uterus is connected to your lower back and your pubic bone by round ligaments. You can imagine that the weight hanging on those round ligaments, which are connected to the bones, can have serious consequences for your body.

You will have certainly felt your pelvis at times during your pregnancy; it might have even caused you real discomfort. Therefore, it makes sense that pelvic issues and round ligament pain are the most common health issues experienced during pregnancy. The good news is you can get rid of these issues through training!

# Pelvic Floor Muscles

The pelvic floor muscles close off the bottom of the pelvis. They are extremely flexible and strong and form a kind of hammock at the bottom of your torso. Those pelvic floor muscles are, as the name suggests, a group of muscles. And just like any other muscle, they can get weaker when they are not trained and too tight when overtrained, and we need them for our body to apply the right force at the right places.

## The Main Functions of Your Pelvic Floor Muscles

- They regulate the opening and closing of the three openings: the urinary tract, vagina, and anus.
- They support the organs: they ensure your organs don't "fall out" at the bottom.
- Your pelvic floor muscles play a major role as a "pump" for your lymphatic system. The better your pelvic floor works, the better the circulation of the lymph fluid.
- They give you (and your partner) sexual pleasure.

## Embarrassment and Pleasure: The Least Normal Muscle Group?

Pelvic floor muscles are simply muscles—and yet, is this muscle group really the same as other muscles?

It is from an anatomical point of view, but from a psychological perspective, this group of muscles is slightly different. You can't see them, and they are in an intimate place on the body that people don't like talking about and are a little embarrassed about. It's a lot easier to say your biceps aren't strong enough and you are going to do some intensive training on them than to say your pelvic floor muscles need a workout. And at what point do you ask your trainer for pelvic floor muscle exercises? Let's be honest, in our head, that muscle group around your vagina and anus is slightly different.

# The Pelvic Floor and Pregnancy

You cannot avoid the fact that your pelvic floor muscles will have suffered a certain amount of "damage" as a result of your pregnancy and the birth, even if you had a cesarean section. During your pregnancy, your pelvic floor muscles became more flexible and softer to enable baby to come out more easily. After childbirth, it's that flexibility and softness that can cause all the trouble. The softer and more flexible the muscles are, the less stability your pelvic floor muscles give you. All those pounds you carried around those nine months also play a part. The more weight you had to carry, the more pressure the pelvic floor muscles had to endure.

How the delivery went also plays a big part in the issues you could have with your pelvic floor muscles after giving birth. If, for instance, you were pushing for a long time, your pelvic floor muscles were under immense pressure for a long time. The movement of the pelvic floor muscles, mainly how much they had to move to allow baby's head to pass through, also influences the amount of "damage" you will have, just as any tear or incision will.

However, you can't say that a woman who pushed for a long time, had an incision, and delivered a baby with a large head will suffer more health issues than a woman who hardly had to push and had a baby with a small head. The condition of your pelvic floor muscles before childbirth also makes a difference. One thing's for sure: the pregnancy and childbirth were an "attack" on your pelvic floor muscles, and that's why you deserve to work on your recovery now.

## FROM BELOW . . . A DETAILED VIEW OF YOUR PELVIC FLOOR MUSCLES

Such a general picture is all well and good, but what do your pelvic floor muscles look like, where are they located, and what do they feel like? Everyone's pelvic floor is unique, and if you get to know yours, you can give this muscle group a better workout. Do the self-test and see how your pelvic floor muscles function on page 260.

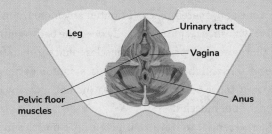

# Rediscover the Connection Between the Pelvic Floor and Brain

Once you have discovered what your pelvic floor muscles look like, how they feel, and their exact position, your brain will need to learn to "rediscover" them. This muscle group has endured a lot, there's a good chance that you are not embracing this part of your body or holding it as dear to your heart as other body parts. Your groin has had a lot to cope with, which often means you sort of mentally distance yourself from your pelvic floor muscles. You may be carrying around that part of your body, but you don't really feel that it is part of you anymore.

You will have to mentally reconnect to your pelvic floor, regain confidence in your pelvic floor, and start to love it again. Okay, that sounds a little vague, but it is perfectly normal that the connection your brain has with those pelvic floor muscles has changed through the pregnancy and childbirth.

That connection is extremely important, however. The more aware you are of these muscles, the easier it will be for you to tighten and relax them and the more naturally it will occur. This will make your recovery quicker, easier, and better. And that's why we start each training session with a specific breathing exercise (XL Breath; see pages 106–107) that includes focusing on your pelvic floor and visualizing how it rises and falls while breathing.

## Crucial: Learning to Tighten and Relax Your Pelvic Floor

People used to believe that the main thing you had to learn after childbirth was how to tighten your pelvic floor muscles again. We know better now. The postpartum programs and standard pelvic floor exercises that are aimed solely at tightening the muscles can actually harm your body. A muscle that is tight all the time and, therefore, can't tighten any more when you really need it (i.e., when you sneeze, jump, or really need the bathroom) is of little use to you. Furthermore, your pelvic floor muscles could become strained and fatigued if they are tense all the time. In fact, most symptoms after pregnancy are caused by overly tense pelvic floor muscles and not, as many believe, by overly slack pelvic floor muscles.

It is, therefore, essential to train your pelvic floor muscles in their "full range of motion." That means from completely relaxed to completely tightened and all "positions" in between.

## Training Pelvic Floor Muscles in a Full Range of Motion:

- Prevents or reduces incontinence
- Prevents prolapses (sagging; see page 36)
- Prevents or reduces pain during intercourse (if not caused by stiff scar tissue in or around the vagina; see page 42)
- Increases your sexual pleasure (your bonus for training: increased sensitivity and more intense orgasms)
- Ensures more moisture production in the vagina
- Contributes to the stability of your powerhouse

## INCONTINENCE: TOO MANY WOMEN SUFFER FROM IT

Incontinence is quite common. Some studies indicate that 30 percent of women have some form of incontinence after childbirth. Others believe that the percentage is even higher, around 50 percent. And then there is the group of women who don't notice it immediately. Symptoms of incontinence don't always appear right away; you might only notice them years later. It is believed that 60 to 80 percent of incontinence issues are caused by pregnancy and childbirth.

### THE RELATIONSHIP BETWEEN LEAKING URINE AND POSTPARTUM DEPRESSION

Women who leak urine involuntarily or have (mild) incontinence are at higher risk of postpartum depression. However, we don't yet know whether there is a direct or indirect link between the two.

# The Pelvic Floor and Abdominal Muscles and the Pressure during Pregnancy

The typical health issues that you might experience in your powerhouse after pregnancy and childbirth are all related to how the pressure was divided in and over the parts of your powerhouse. During your pregnancy, there was a type of battle going on between the pressure from the abdominal cavity and the strength of your muscles. If your muscles are too weak or the parts of your powerhouse don't function properly as a whole, the excessive pressure from the abdominal cavity could become so great that you could get a hernia (usually at the top), diastasis recti (centrally over the belly), or a prolapse (sagging of the underside). See it this way: if the pressure builds up and it cannot be released to the back, through your spine, then it must escape another way: outward or downward.

## Hernia

A hernia occurs when a specific part of your body that resides in the abdominal cavity comes out at the weakest part of your abdominal wall. A hernia can occur at any weak point, but during pregnancy it is usually at your belly button. Suddenly there is a small bulge at that small hole where your belly button was. It's actually fine and certainly not serious. However, it indicates a weak spot in your body where the pressure in the abdominal cavity has built up to such a degree that it caused the belly button to pop out. It usually plops back in after childbirth and sometimes even during the final weeks of pregnancy because baby descends and the shape of the belly changes, and that changes the pressure on certain places in the belly. Navel hernias (*hernia umbilicus*) are quite common and not serious. A naval hernia only becomes an issue if it doesn't get better after childbirth or if it reoccurs after childbirth. In that case, it is advisable to tackle that weak spot to avoid surgery. You do that by making sure your abdominal muscles function properly (that they are strong but also that they are functioning as they are supposed to) and by paying attention to your posture. That latter is often still underestimated!

# IF YOU ARE URINATING FREQUENTLY

You will have certainly needed the bathroom a lot more than usual when you were pregnant. It's a logical consequence of the increased pressure on your bladder and less space in your abdomen. But what if that frequent urination continues after childbirth? First, check whether there's any obvious reason. For example, are you drinking a lot more because you are breast-feeding, or could you have a bladder infection? If you can't find an apparent reason, then you need to do something about it. Consult your physician.

## DR. SONIA BAHLANI, gynecologist, New York, USA

Many women who have suffer with "frequent urination" still too often hear that it's part of having a child. It's not part of it. And waiting six months for it to pass isn't the ideal option either. You have enough to do as a mother as it is, and when you finally get to sleep, you don't want to be woken up by your bladder.

If there is no obvious reason, then the first thing you should do is figure out why you need to urinate so often.

1. Could your pelvic floor muscles be too tight? When you urinate, the bladder contracts and presses the urine out, as it were. Your pelvic floor muscles relax and open so that the urine can exit through the urinary tract. But if your pelvic floor muscles can't relax properly, they cramp up and close off the flow of urine too soon. The result is you don't empty your bladder completely and you will need to go to the bathroom more often. And this has consequences for infections. Infections can get worse if you don't empty your bladder. It is therefore important to do good pelvic floor muscle exercises that also focus on relaxing them.

2. Another option is treating the so-called trigger points in your vagina (see page 143). Seeing as the pelvic floor muscle is a muscle, it can get "knotted." By treating and loosening the knots, your pelvic floor muscles will not cramp as soon as they are touched (e.g., due to the pressure of the flow of urine or penetration). Once the knot has been loosened, it is important it stays that way. A natural muscle relaxant such as magnesium or valerian tea often achieves that.

3. There are times when that is not enough, and you need medical intervention. There are medicines that help your muscles relax and that are safe to use when breastfeeding. Some drugs are taken orally, but there are also injections that can help the muscles relax.

Adopting a good posture decreases the pressure on your abdominal cavity. Try it: when you lean forward, everything in your belly is "crushed," which is not the case when you literally give it space by sitting up straight. The same applies to standing. If the pressure in your abdominal cavity is getting too much, it is even more important to literally give your belly space by adopting a good straight posture (see page 94).

## Diastasis (Diastasis Recti)

Your vertical and oblique abdominal muscles form a lovely corset around your belly, keeping everything in place, giving you strength, and helping maintain your posture. During the second or third trimester of your pregnancy, your vertical abdominal muscles (or your "six-pack" abdominal muscles) in particular move to accommodate the growth of your uterus. These muscles normally run from under your breastbone straight down to your pubic bone. The two straight abdominal muscles are connected to each other by a thick strip of connective tissue (the linea alba). When you are not pregnant, the linea alba is roughly a finger wide. When you are pregnant, the influence of hormones and particularly the internal pressure make the muscles and connective tissue more flexible, and the vertical muscles move farther away from each other. They are still connected by the linea alba. The abdominal muscles don't become completely separated or split as we often hear. It is only the connection between the two muscles that stretches: the diastasis increases.

It is normal for the space between the abdominal muscles to widen, for example, from ½ to 1 inch. Usually, the linea alba goes back to normal by itself within six months after childbirth. If the diastasis is larger than 1 inch, it might not return by itself. That used to mean surgery. Fortunately, opinions have changed, and the current advice is to see whether a woman can first reduce the diastasis herself through the right exercises.

Nowadays, we also know that as well as checking the width of the diastasis, we need to look at how firm the linea alba is. You want it to feel strong and rubbery.

It is important to reduce the diastasis, not only for your core strength but also because 66 percent of women with a large diastasis develop pelvic floor issues as a result. In short, you have very good reasons to give those vertical abdominal muscles a workout!

You can see it this way: if your vertical abdominal muscles are the front facade of your powerhouse, when you have a large diastasis it is as if your door or windows are wide open. The BTY program ensures your front facade can close properly once more. Do the self-test on page 261.

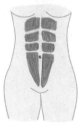
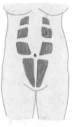
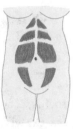
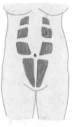
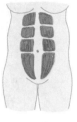

| Normal diastasis | Open diastasis | Open diastasis below the navel | Open diastasis above the navel | Completely open diastasis |

## YOU HAVE AN INCREASED CHANCE OF DEVELOPING DIASTASIS RECTI WHEN:

- You were over 34 years during your pregnancy.
- You have given birth to a big baby.
- You had a lot of amniotic fluid.
- You had multiple births.
- You have been pregnant before.
- Before this pregnancy, you had a baby by cesarean section.
- You suffered from increased pressure in your belly (e.g., because you breathe "high up" in your body, thereby increasing the pressure on your midriff).
- You have suffered or are suffering badly from constipation.
- You are slim or have thin skin (the diastasis often occurs around or just above the belly button).

## EVERYONE HAS A DIASTASIS

The linea alba is made to stretch, and that happens during pregnancy, of course. That is a diastasis, but there's no need to be alarmed. Just as the linea alba is made to stretch, it is also made to return to its former shape. A diastasis is, therefore, completely normal and part of pregnancy and childbirth. It only causes health conditions, problems, and restrictions if the diastasis is too large or the linea alba is too weak. When people talk about diastasis recti, it is often used to mean an extreme type of diastasis.

## YOU CAN DO THE FOLLOWING IF YOU HAVE A (LARGE) DIASTASIS OR (WEAK) LINEA ALBA

You can do this yourself:

- **Watch your posture.** Yes, there it is again, that posture! But it really is that important. With the wrong posture, the abdominal muscles come under more pressure, and right now they can't cope with any more. Avoid stretching the vertical abdominal muscles to the max. Don't slouch forward, especially not with your arms up, because then you extend the vertical abdominal muscles, and you should avoid that now.

- **Stay active.** It will only get worse if you don't move enough. Tissue and therefore also muscles only improve when they come under pressure or, in other words, when they move or are trained.

- **A specialized pelvic floor therapist can help you by applying tape to give specific external support.** This is often done in the first phase of recovery, and it will also teach you about adopting a good posture in the midriff region. A specialist knows exactly what to do and will provide the right level of support. It will not be too little but not too much, either, because too much support can make your muscles lazy and weak.

## THIS IS HOW THE BTY PROGRAM CAN HELP REDUCE YOUR DIASTASIS

- **We train the other abdominal muscles, such as the deep transverse abdominal muscles, a bit harder** because these stabilize your core without overburdening your vertical abdominal muscles.

- **We encourage stretching and prevent you from overstretching.** You must avoid overstretching your vertical abdominal muscles so that they can go back together. Our exercises are designed so that you can't overstretch them. We do stretch the surrounding muscles, though. We do that because these muscles often overcompensate for the inactive abdominal muscles. Because the abdominal muscles are not functioning perfectly right now, the surrounding muscles start working overtime and therefore cramp. That is why we stretch them, and we do all we can to help you regain the right balance.

- **Avoid such exercises as crunches and sit-ups until the "You" phase and while your diastasis is large or your linea alba is still weak.** Don't worry; when you are going through the BTY program, we ask you to check your diastasis regularly, and the exercises are geared to your personal recovery.

- **Do gentle rotating exercises and exercises on all fours.** The exercises make sure that you won't be caught off guard in daily life. People used to assume that you shouldn't sit on your hands and knees or rotate (twist) your middle when you have a large diastasis. That opinion has changed. There's no doubt that this position and movement are hard work for your abdominal muscles, but these types of movements are difficult to avoid in daily life. At some point, we all change our baby's diaper on hands and knees on the floor. And we all grab things while twisting our body on occasion. When you have not trained your body to make these movements, they will be even harder for you. It is, therefore, better to do training exercises so that you control the position and movement rather than giving your body a shock. The training we do in these hand-knee positions and the rotating movements are gentle, and we gradually build them up.

- **Watch out for gravity.** If you have a very large diastasis, you should be careful with exercises where gravity pushes down on these abdominal muscles—in short, exercises where you lean forward. You don't have to avoid them completely, but be careful and stop if you feel discomfort or pain (other than "normal workout pain"). We will, of course, warn you when we ask you to do these types of exercises in the BTY program.

## DR. JUDITH MEER, PT, DPT, CSCS,
### pelvic floor therapist, New Jersey, USA

Many women are unaware that therapists can treat diastasis recti in various ways and not only by prescribing exercises. For example, I use a myofascial release technique that releases muscle knots and reduces skin tension to relieve restrictions in the back, loins, and abdomen that arose as the belly grew during pregnancy. This can help to bring the sides of the abdominal muscles back together. I often apply several pieces of elastic kinesiology tape to the upper body; the tape can stay in place while the patient goes about her daily activities. Keep in mind that the tips you find online about how to tape your abdominal wall are not geared to your personal situation. In general, they are less effective than if you consult a good physiotherapist who can evaluate your personal restrictions and tape them correctly. If, for example, you tend to carry your baby on your left side, that will cause more tension on the tissue on that side of your body. This means that the tape should be applied so that there is more "pulling force" from the left to the right side. If this technique is properly applied by an experienced therapist, an eight-finger-wide diastasis can be reduced to three fingers within a few treatments. It may sound incredible, but I've seen it happen!

## Prolapse (Sagging)

When the pelvic floor is not functioning as it should (you can't tighten it at the right times, it's too weak or too tense), the pelvic organs could fall out of place or sag. A weak pelvic floor isn't always to blame for a prolapse, however. After all, your pelvic floor is not the only body part responsible for keeping everything inside. The rest of your powerhouse also plays a significant role.

Prolapses are more common than you might think. There are experts who estimate that half of women have a form of prolapse after pregnancy, and about a quarter suffer from a prolapse for the rest of their life to a greater or lesser degree. And yet hardly anyone talks about it. Some women don't even realize they have a prolapse, and others believe it's normal following childbirth. As to the issue of whether it's normal, well, it's common but it's certainly not normal, and you don't have to suffer from the consequences for the rest of your life. That is, if you do the right training and exercises and start early enough. The first two degrees of prolapse can be corrected with training and help. It's a lot harder if you have (or wait until you have) a stage three or four prolapse.

**STAGE 1:** You have a mild prolapse; it doesn't cause any real symptoms and that's why you often don't even notice you have it unless you check yourself regularly.

**STAGE 2:** There is a notable protrusion below; however, nothing comes through the opening of the vagina when you push.

**STAGE 3:** When you push, something protrudes out of the opening of the vagina.

**STAGE 4:** The prolapse now comes out of the vagina without your pushing.

Do the self-test on page 264 to see whether you have the symptoms of a prolapse.

## DR. SHEILA DE LIZ, gynecologist, Wiesbaden, Germany

Don't delay in getting a checkup if you think you could have a prolapse. Stages one and two can be helped through exercise, but three and four often need to be corrected with surgery. It's good this option exists, but it's not the ideal situation. One of the problems of the surgery is how the entire clitoris and all the feeling recover afterward. If you are unlucky enough to need this surgery, make sure it is carried out by a surgeon who will take that into account.

## YOU CAN DO THE FOLLOWING WHEN YOU HAVE A PROLAPSE

Do this yourself:
- **Watch your posture when standing and sitting.** The same applies here as with a hernia: if you stand or sit hunched over, your abdominal cavity has less space, which increases the pressure on the pelvic floor muscles even more. See pages 97 and 98.
- **Watch your sitting posture when going to the bathroom (see page 103).** Well, it may sound a little crazy, but you demand a whole lot of your pelvic floor when you use the toilet, especially when pushing (and you shouldn't do that).

- **Inserting a diaphragm (cervical cap) can help sometimes.** Contact your family physician about it.
- **Never push!** When you push, you hold in your breath, causing the pressure to build up in your belly. You turn that pressure into force that you put on the lower part of your body. That is the last thing you want when you have a prolapse. Therefore, never push. Not when going to the bathroom, or when lifting something heavy or doing strenuous movements. Don't be tempted to push just that one time. Even pushing once will set you right back in your recovery. Pay special attention to your breathing. Keep it regulated and exhale normally.

## THIS IS HOW THE BTY PROGRAM CAN HELP YOU REDUCE YOUR PROLAPSE

- We train your pelvic floor muscles to get rid of your prolapse.
- We train your entire powerhouse because it can compensate for your weak spot.
- We avoid exercises that increase the pressure too much, and we do them in an effective mini version (e.g., we train your buttocks using mini squats). Your pelvis gains stability through the connection with your butt muscles. You reap double the benefits from strong buttocks. Really pay attention to your breathing because if you push to do the mini squat you will build up internal pressure, which will only make the prolapse worse!

## PRESSURE DISTRIBUTION: THE KEY TO GOOD RECOVERY

Almost all issues in your powerhouse come from incorrect pressure distribution. The key to a good recovery is in spreading out that pressure. All our training, posture, and breathing exercises are based on distributing the pressure. The better distributed it is, the better it is for your powerhouse.

# Everything Is Connected: The Domino Effect

The central position of your powerhouse means that specific posture issues can affect many other body parts. This is the so-called domino effect. For example, you could get a headache due to walking lopsided to reduce round ligament pain during the pregnancy. And it can also work the other way around: incorrect foot positioning can influence your hips, causing you to tilt them inward or outward when walking. That tilting of the hips reduces the amount of space in the abdominal cavity, putting your powerhouse under more pressure than necessary. Don't worry; we will tackle your whole body and mind with your personal BTY program.

# YOU AND
# YOUR VAGINA

That wonderful spot *down below*. That part where you can feel exceptional pleasure, that part where you feel arousal, and that part where,
if you had a vaginal birth, you pushed out an entire person. Even if you gave
birth by cesarean section, your vagina had a whole lot to endure because
of the pressure it was under. Let's be honest, there's a big chance that your
vagina doesn't feel or look the same as it did before. It's time to turn the tide
and start enjoying everything this exceptional body part can do again. We
are living in the 21st century, after all ;-).

## DID YOU GIVE BIRTH OVER EIGHT WEEKS AGO?

If so, the followings symptoms are not normal in your vagina
(and don't be mistaken; many women have one or more of these
symptoms).

- Burning sensation (often after urinating or after
  penetrative sex)
- Pain or a feeling of discomfort
- Odors
- Pain if you sit down for a long time
- Pain during penetration or in certain positions

See your family physician, gynecologist, or pelvic floor therapist if
you have any of these symptoms.

# Your Vagina: No Pain and No Discomfort

It makes sense that your vagina needs to heal and recover from childbirth
in the first weeks. After about six to eight weeks, your vagina has usually
recovered in a medical sense, and you should be able to do all the things you
used to do—things ranging from inserting a tampon to masturbating and
the thing that started this whole journey of pregnancy and recovery: sex.

And yet, that purely medical recovery is not all it's cracked up to be. After
six to eight weeks, you could have a full and lovely sex life, but that is seldom
the case. Apart from a few exceptions, you couldn't really call the first year
after childbirth the highpoint of your sex life. And that is not surprising
because . . .

- You could have scars (physical).
- The pH level in your vagina changes, resulting in dryness (physical).
- The feeling in your vagina has changed (physical).
- You may be anxious about putting something inside your vagina after pushing out something so big (emotional).
- Your priorities could have changed (emotional).
- The way you see yourself could have changed (emotional).
- You may look at your partner differently now (relational).

No matter how logical these things are, a few simple adjustments can bring back your desire to have sex or even make it better than it ever was. Let's bring that sex(y) back!

## AND . . . WHEN CAN YOU HAVE SEX AGAIN?

You can have sex when you are ready for it and it's medically responsible. And that varies for each woman. You have an increased risk of infection before the bleeding stops because the cervix isn't completely closed. And that's why you are advised to wait to have penetrative sex until the bleeding has stopped, or only have sex with a condom. During your postpartum checkup, you will be examined to see whether everything has fully recovered and whether it's safe to have sex.

## What's the Deal with My Scars?

Many women tear during childbirth or have an incision, and that tear or incision causes a temporary wound. You will be examined during your final postpartum checkup to see whether it has completely healed. When it has, you'll know that it's safe to put pressure on that area without you tearing again. But let's be honest, knowing and believing are two different things. Furthermore, your body could be telling you other things than the medics can. You can feel the scars, which could make it harder to believe that it's all okay again.

It can help to see what the scars look like. Grab a hand mirror and look at your scars. You will see they are a lot calmer and look better than you thought. Can you see them? Yes, you can. They are scars, after all, and they need time to become less noticeable. Also look at the area around the scars because you will also notice a difference there. Compare it to a T-shirt: if it's torn and you stitch it closed, the area around the repair will wrinkle up.

Fortunately, vaginal tissue is more forgiving and doesn't wrinkle, but that's not to say that the area around the scar will not have been affected.

Massage your scar tissue! See page 178.

## The pH Level in Your Vagina Changes and Your Vagina May Become Drier

It's not common knowledge, but it's so important to know that even the acid level, the pH value, in your vagina changes in the period after childbirth. You may have noticed that your vagina is drier than normal and that it smells differently.

In turn, that dryness can cause all kinds of health issues, such as:

- (Recurring) vaginal infections
- A burning sensation
- Pain during sex
- Changes to the way or how frequently you urinate

### DR. SONIA BAHLANI, gynecologist, New York, USA

You shouldn't put up with all these types of symptoms, and you don't have to. All too often, people around you, and even physicians sometimes, say it's all part of childbirth and that it will eventually pass. But why wait? Why should you accept the pain and discomfort when you don't have to? In fact, if you don't do anything about the pain, it will only get worse.

See your physician if you have any of these symptoms and push the point. Don't let them brush you off. There are various options from a medical perspective, but there are also natural substances, such as natural organic lubricants. Try them. It won't do any harm to give them a go! (Do not, however, use butter, spit, or baby oil.) It appears that a daily supplement of 1,000 IU of vitamin $D_3$ can also have a positive effect on the pH level in the vagina.

Some drugs, such as antidepressants, can worsen such issues as a dry vagina or a lack of passion and make reaching an orgasm even more difficult. It could be a good idea to check whether you still really need the drugs or see whether they can be replaced by something else. Estriol cream, which is only available by doctor's prescription, can be a great help if your vagina is very dry.

## Where Has All the Feeling Gone?

There is a chance your vagina is less sensitive. It all seems slightly numb and more spacious to start with. That spaciousness will gradually lessen, and it will tighten up again; the exercises will help with that. But until then, you could pass "vaginal wind." There is whole lot of extra space in your vagina, which fills with air, and that air needs to escape. As your vagina becomes tighter, the vaginal wind will pass, and the feeling will increasingly return.

There are actually two types of feeling in your vagina: the one that helps you to reach an orgasm and the one you feel when lightly touched. With that first type, you need your muscles to contract together during an orgasm. And then we are talking about—here they are again—the pelvic floor muscles. With the second type of sensation, it is more about the feeling of touching the skin of the vagina. That skin was stretched and was under extreme pressure during childbirth. That applies more to women who gave birth vaginally, but it also applies to women who had a cesarean section. The feeling and the nerves in the skin need to recover. Blood flow also plays a big part here. The better the blood flow to the skin, the more you feel. And you can help that blood flow improve.

## HELP THE BLOOD FLOW IN YOUR VAGINA AND CLITORIS

- **There are natural organic oils that stimulate blood flow.**
  Apply the oil to your clitoris and the area around your vagina 15 to 30 minutes before having sex. You will soon notice that it all becomes more sensitive. If you use condoms, make sure you use condoms that work with oil-based lubricants.

- **There are also lubricants that stimulate blood flow.** Choose a natural, organic, water-based variety, one that doesn't contain silicones, and don't insert anything that could negatively affect the pH level of your vagina. Also, be careful with lubricants before the skin in and around the vagina is completely healed. Whatever lubricant you choose, make sure to read first about any possible side effects.

## Something Has to Go in Where?

Apart from the physical changes to your vagina, the emotional side also plays a part, especially if childbirth didn't go smoothly. The thought of something entering your vagina could be a very scary one. It makes perfect sense, but you can help your body by getting over this fear.

Be aware that almost all women find sex scary the first time after childbirth, and their partners often do, too. Take your time. Cuddle lots, massage each other, and don't see sex only as penetration. It can be just as lovely to look deep into your partner's eyes, lie in their wonderful arms, and enjoy the sensation of a hand running over your body while you completely surrender to the calming feeling. You can fully relax, go to a place deep inside yourself "as a woman," and forget the rest of the world. Oxytocin, "the love hormone," will run through your entire body, and that relaxes you. It could even be so relaxing that it leads to penetration. It could feel strange, different, or even slightly painful the first time, but by using a lubricant, there's a big chance you'll feel less discomfort because it will go more smoothly.

## THIS IS HOW TO REGAIN CONFIDENCE IN YOUR VAGINA

1. You can regain confidence in penetration by feeling inside your vagina, using a clean finger, for example, to see what it's like to have something inside it. Try to "embrace" your fingers with your pelvic floor by tensing the muscles. Concentrate on the feeling in your entire vagina. Notice how it works, feel what it does, and you'll realize it's all okay.
2. Sex with your partner is one thing, but you can also regain confidence in your body by masturbating. Do what feels nice for

you, whether that is stroking yourself with your hand or using pressure from a dildo to arouse yourself, for example. As long as you enjoy it and it helps your confidence, it's all good (and nice ;-)). If you don't enjoy it that much, you could try applying an oil that stimulates blood flow before masturbating. If you can't reach orgasm, don't make a big deal of it. Right now, it's all about regaining confidence in your vagina and the fact something can penetrate it again without you being anxious.

3. There are cases when a woman is unable to handle penetration by her own finger or a dildo, and some feel nothing at all can enter their vagina, not even a pinkie finger. It is as if their vagina is locked down. If that is the case, a vaginal dilator could be a solution. First apply a lubricant and put the smallest part of the dilator inside your vagina, then slowly increase the size. If this causes you issues, it's highly advisable to see a pelvic specialist.

## DID YOU KNOW THAT . . .

Your breasts can leak or even spray milk when you orgasm? The hormone oxytocin is released during an orgasm. It works as a let-down reflex, which means your body could see that shot of oxytocin as a sign to let the breast milk flow.

### Sex or Romance? Well, That's Not High on My List of Priorities Right Now . . .

You have a lot to cope with as a new mom. You "must" do all sorts of things, you get all types of new impressions, have sleepless nights, are worrying about this and that, are feeling the pressure of a chronic lack of time, and you can't even remember how to spell the word *romance*. Amid all these life-changing emotions, sex is not on your list of priorities. It's perfectly logical. But still . . . it's a shame!

Of course, you shouldn't have sex if you are not in the mood for it. But sex is part of a healthy relationship. Talk to your partner about it, avoid feelings of rejection or insecurity from coming up. It will keep your relationship healthy until you are both in the mood to have some lovely sex.

## ANN-MARLENE HENNING, sex and relationship therapist, Hamburg, Germany

There is a model in sexology, the *dual control model*, which assumes that all people have sexual excitation and inhibition. Or put simply: gas and brakes. The most notable recent knowledge about this is that they both work and are present at the same time. The desire to have sex is thus the result of a continuous interaction between the two. Some people have more gas than brakes, and others have more brakes. This can be compared to being extroverted or introverted: it's not learned behavior but how you are. Sexual excitation and inhibition have a substantial influence on you and are inherently linked to your development as a sexual being. Motherhood can easily become a "brake" for people with many inhibitions. You can't change your innate "gas and brakes," but you can change the way you deal with them. Be aware of this, and don't let your maternal feelings stand in the way of a good sex life.

## THE VAGINA: A PIGGY BANK FOR TRAUMAS AND EMOTIONS?

It has not been proven (yet), but it seems that the vagina holds on to unprocessed emotions, as it were. Those emotions can vary from a trauma during childbirth to unprocessed emotions from long ago. Some researchers even believe this is one of the causes of vaginismus, whereby the vagina spasms so strongly that penetration, even with a finger or tampon, is impossible. This once again shows how your mind and body are so intrinsically linked. Sometimes you must work on one to help the other.

### Your Relationship May Have Changed

No matter how well and how long you have known each other, or how much you wanted children together, you could find yourself suddenly seeing your partner in a different light or realizing that your partner sees you differently now. Having a child is life changing for both of you.

You are both reborn, in a way: from a woman to a (co-)mother, from a man to a father. This is also an opportunity for you to rediscover each other and to get to know each other again in your new roles. It isn't always all romance, though; you could notice that you no longer feel the way you did before, or you think your partner feels differently. Talk about it. Make sure you don't lose each other. If you can't sort it out together, then get help from a relationship therapist. You'd be surprised how many new families take this step. Parenthood is no mean feat, after all!

## Everything Works, but I'm Simply Not in the Mood

There are times when the problem is not pain, unease, confidence, anxieties, priorities, or your relationship. You could simply not be in the mood for sex. Listen to how you feel, but if you used to have a good and enjoyable sex life, then deep down you will be secretly missing it a little. If you feel that it is taking too long for your libido to return, then see your physician, a pelvic therapist, or a sexologist.

## HOW DOES AN ORGASM OCCUR?

We have all had them at some point (hopefully), but how does an orgasm work, exactly? And did you know that your clitoris is bigger than that one small bobble? And did you know that there are four ways to orgasm and that the exercises in the BTY program can also help you have better and more intense orgasms?

### FOUR TYPES OF ORGASMS

**1. THE CLITORAL ORGASM:** Without a doubt, the clitoris is the most sensitive part of the female body. But the clitoris is much bigger than that little bobble we feel. The clitoris runs along the outside of your vagina, which makes the entire area extremely sensitive. Because all 8,000 (!) nerves come together at the bobble, the rest of the clitoris seems less sensitive. But 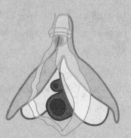 you shouldn't dismiss the power of the rest. By stimulating the other parts of the clitoris first (along the vagina wall and above the bobble) and waiting before touching the most sensitive part, your orgasm will be more intense when you do stimulate it.

**2. THE VAGINAL ORGASM:** You can also orgasm by stimulating the inside of the vagina. Search for that sensitive spot: the G-spot. You can find it on the inside of your vagina, up about 2 inches at the back of your clitoris. In the world of sexual orgasm research, there is an ongoing discussion as to whether the G-spot is a separate organ or part of the clitoris. Well, whether it's a separate part or the end of another part, we know that if you can find it you can have very full and intense vaginal orgasms. The G-spot feels spongy, ribbed, and it fills up with fluid the more aroused you become. By changing positions and feeling when the penis or dildo touches that wonderful spot, you can discover exactly where your G-spot is. But even when you have found it, a vaginal orgasm is often harder to achieve than a clitoral orgasm.

**3. BLENDED ORGASM:** A vaginal and clitoral orgasm at the same time is called a blended orgasm. Women who have experienced this know that it's more than two types of orgasm at the same time: it is 1 + 1 = 3 orgasms. It can't get more intense than that. You can have this type of orgasm by sitting on top of your partner. Turn until you feel they are touching your G-spot, and when you or your partner stimulates the most sensitive part of the clitoris, you have a good chance of having a blended orgasm.

**4. MULTIPLE ORGASMS:** When you are having a long lovemaking session, you could orgasm several times. Then we're talking about multiple orgasms. The more often you have sex, the easier it is to have multiple orgasms.

## WHAT IS AN ORGASM, EXACTLY?

During that moment of ultimate pleasure, all the pelvic floor muscles and the rear of the vagina rhythmically contract together. They contract, relax, contract again and relax again, and so on. The better you can contract your muscles and then relax them, the more intense your orgasm will be. To put it simply, an orgasm is a muscle movement. The better trained the muscle is, the better it works. Therefore, the pelvic floor exercises not only have medical benefits; they have other nice benefits as well.

Your interest in sex is a significant measure of your health.

—DR. JOLENE BRIGHTEN, naturopathic physician, biochemist, and expert in female hormones, Seattle, USA

# 10 Benefits of Sex for Women

1. It is good for your immune system! When you have sex more than once a week, you have more immunoglobin A. This fights off a range of pathogens.
2. It boosts your serotonin levels: the neurotransmitter that gives you "happy feelings."
3. It lowers your blood pressure, which is good for your cardiovascular system (circulatory system).
4. It reduces stress. Your cortisol (stress hormone) levels decrease, and you get a boost of dopamine right in the part of the brain that makes you feel satisfied and rewarded.
5. It helps you relax and sleep. When you orgasm, you release a whole lot of prolactin, allowing you to relax and fall asleep.
6. Sex actually exercises your pelvic floor muscles! Every time you make love, this special group of muscles gets an extra workout.
7. It improves brain function . . . in the long term, in any case. Women who have sex regularly during their lifetime will benefit in the cognitive part of their brain.
8. Sex devours calories, making it the most enjoyable fat-burning workout there is.
9. Sex is good for your self-confidence. Your self-confidence grows when you feel loved, and you radiate that. Self-confidence attracts others and draws people to you, so your self-confidence increases further. In short, a wonderful upward spiral.
10. Sex is good for your relationship.

# YOU AND YOUR HORMONES

During your pregnancy, there would have been no escaping that your body and mood were affected by your hormones. We all know that hormones can cause issues when you have your period. Less is known about the role of hormones during postpartum recovery. In fact, almost all aspects of recovery after childbirth and many things that seem to be "purely" physical are influenced by your hormones. From the baby blues to dryness in your vagina . . . blame the hormones. There you were, thinking you were done with them after childbirth, and you have to get used to new hormone levels all over again.

## WHY LEARN ALL ABOUT HORMONES?

You could say you are recovered when your body has recovered, found its old strength, and when you have gotten used to your new hormone levels. You can help and accelerate that process of adjustment through your lifestyle choices. Are you helping your body or working against it? To understand the effect of your choices, and because you might find it interesting, here we first explain what hormones are, how they work, and how they affect your postpartum recovery.

# What Are Hormones?

Hormones are actually messengers carrying information that tells specific cells what to do. They are made by glands, and they travel though the body via the bloodstream. Hormones play a vital role in almost every process that takes place in our body. These range from the sleeping-waking rhythm, to maintaining a constant body temperature, to regulating blood sugar levels, to the amount of urine produced, to repairing wounds, to fighting infections, and the list could go on for pages. The short version is, when our hormone levels are off-balance, it has a major impact on our body and our mind. We are discovering more and more about hormones, particularly in relation to postpartum recovery. Recent studies have shown, for example, that there is a direct link between hormones and postpartum depression and even incontinence.

# These Hormones Play a Role after Childbirth

Okay, so those hormones control everything in a way. But which hormones are we talking about and what do they do, exactly?

## Estrogen

The word *estrogen* suggests one hormone, but we should actually say estrogens because we are dealing with a club of three hormones, each with its own function: estradiol (function: fertility and bone density), estriol (mainly produced during pregnancy), and estrone (mainly produced in the fatty tissue after menopause).

Furthermore, this hormone helps you produce endorphin, a sort of "feel good" substance. Endorphins influence your mood and have a pain-relieving effect. This has rightly earned them the title of "your body's morphine."

## Oxytocin

Oxytocin is also called the "cuddle hormone." Everyone produces oxytocin during positive mutual contact. That includes when cuddling and during sex, and with intense eye contact. The production of oxytocin makes you feel more safe and secure. This hormone, therefore, plays a major role in developing a very special bond with your baby.

Right after childbirth, the uterus starts contracting under the influence of oxytocin: the postpartum contractions. This allows your womb to regain its former, smaller size. During those contractions, the torn blood vessels are pulled closer together and thus squeezed closed. Oxytocin is, therefore, partly responsible for stopping the uterus from bleeding.

Oxytocin's second role is during breastfeeding. It is not that breast milk is made under the influence of this hormone, but oxytocin ensures its supply in the form of the let-down reflex.

## Adrenaline and Cortisol

Adrenaline and cortisol are two different stress hormones. And don't be mistaken; stress isn't always a bad thing. Sometimes your body needs a signal to give your all, be alert, and go beyond your boundaries. Consider if you need to flee suddenly or must do something extremely difficult that you would give up on without adrenaline in your system—for instance, childbirth. Sometimes you really need that extra dose of adrenaline and/or cortisol; and at other times, you don't. Fortunately, oxytocin inhibits the production of adrenaline at the right times.

If life is getting on top of you or you feel down, you produce excessive amounts of adrenaline and cortisol. Your body is continually weighed down by stress, which again affects your hormone levels and, therefore, your state of mind. Your state of mind is influenced by the amount of cortisol in your body. That cortisol sharpens your senses, meaning you experience the world more intensely and strongly.

It gets even worse if the period of stress lasts for a long time and the adrenal glands, which produce the anti-inflammatory cortisol, become exhausted and stop producing enough cortisol. People faced with this are reaching a burnout. They are often incapable of processing stimuli, and everything gets to be too much. You often see that these people get sick often and easily.

Therefore, rest is an essential element to ensure good hormonal balance.

Furthermore, high levels of adrenaline in your body ensure that your testosterone levels drop.

In short, stress has a function, but long-term stress works against your body and your recovery.

## Testosterone

Testosterone is a typical male hormone, but don't be mistaken—women produce it, too. And that's a good thing because, combined with estrogen and progesterone, it forms the basis for things like good muscle mass, stimulates the libido, gives you energy, and makes you more assertive.

You always produce testosterone, whether pregnant or not. With the right level of high-intensity interval training (HIIT) and strength training, you can produce testosterone in a highly effective manner.

## Human Growth Hormone (HGH)

As the name suggests, this hormone's job includes making new muscle cells and bone tissue. Furthermore, this hormone ensures that the body contains the right amount of fat, water, and muscle. You need this hormone during your recovery to allow your muscles to grow, to recover, and, indirectly, to lose weight.

## Prolactin

After childbirth, prolactin encourages milk production. Each time you breast-feed, this hormone has a kind of peak in production so that you produce enough milk for the following feed. That's why it's advisable to continue feeding throughout the night, and partly because the prolactin level in your blood is at its highest at night and in the early morning. Once milk production is well underway, this hormone's role decreases and breastfeeding is regulated locally.

## DR. JOLENE BRIGHTEN, naturopathic physician, biochemist, and female hormone expert, Seattle, USA

Ideally, you should have a peak of cortisol in the morning. That level should decrease throughout the day and be low in the evening, while your melatonin levels should be high. That makes you calm, and you will be able to sleep well. We often notice that mothers with a baby have high levels of cortisol that don't drop in the evenings. That has a negative effect on the brain. The brain can recover from the day when melatonin levels are high at night and cortisol levels are low. That doesn't work optimally if cortisol levels are too high. It is also harder to rest properly when your cortisol levels are too high throughout the day rather than just peaking in the morning. If you are not well rested, that can, in turn, cause headaches and the like.

### MY TIPS:

- **Eat regularly and drink plenty.** It sounds pretty straightforward, but it's especially important. Dehydration causes stress and irregular blood sugar levels.
- **Go outside first thing in the morning** or, in any case, make sure you get a lot of daylight. This encourages the production of the normal levels of cortisol in the morning and breaks down the melatonin you still have in your blood from the night before.
- **Consider taking *Rhodiola rosea* (a.k.a. rose root) to stimulate your stamina.** Or opt for licorice root in the morning. But watch out; you shouldn't consume it if you have high blood pressure. Licorice root ensures that the little bit of cortisol stays around throughout the day. If you don't produce a good peak of cortisol, it can help you peak a little longer. Or, in other words, you won't be as tired and you will be better able to get through the day.

## Relaxin

The name will have given away that this hormone has something to do with relaxation. And that's correct, although it's mainly about a physical form of relaxation. When you were pregnant, relaxin worked alongside progesterone to loosen your joints, pelvic ligaments, and cervix (they became even more relaxed). This made it easier for you to deliver your baby. It's one of Mother Nature's clever devices, but it does have disadvantages. The hormone relaxin is not only present in your pelvic area but in your entire body. In short, all your joints have become more supple, and that can cause balance and stability issues. Once you have given birth, the high levels of relaxin in your blood rapidly decrease. But that doesn't suddenly get rid of these balance and stability issues. Now that your pregnancy is over, the weaker body parts need to regain their former strength so that you regain your former stability.

# From a Major Increase during Pregnancy to a Drastic Drop after the Delivery

Your body is made to produce the right hormones at the right time. In fact, certain signals cause a massive dose of a specific hormone to be made immediately—you could almost say, from one second to the next. If you get a fright, then a massive dose of adrenaline is instantly released. When the sperm cell penetrates the egg cell and pregnancy occurs, the body immediately adjusts all the hormone levels so that the fertilized egg cell has a chance to nestle and develop. It is that sudden change that can make the hormones hard to cope with. The change is so sudden, your body doesn't have a chance to gradually get used to it. It is suddenly confronted with totally different levels than ever before. That sudden increase in estrogens is one of the reasons you had numerous ailments in the first weeks of your pregnancy. Later in the pregnancy, you had a massive increase in progesterone levels, which slackened your body and, in turn, caused all kinds of symptoms.

It's not that different just before labor starts. Just before your contractions begin, the estrogen level shoots up again.

Your hormone levels change even more drastically when you release the placenta. That excessively high level of progesterone you produced during the pregnancy drops within a few hours to almost the same level as before the pregnancy. You could say your body wants to regain its natural menstrual cycle as quickly as possible. That doesn't mean, however, that you will have your period again soon because that is inhibited by the hormone prolactin, which you produce when breastfeeding.

It's pretty much the same with the estrogens. Within a few days to weeks after childbirth, the estrogen levels go from sky high to the level you had prior to pregnancy. Therefore, within a few days, your body has completely different hormone levels compared to those it had during the pregnancy. You had just gotten used to the new pregnancy hormones and it all kicks off again. Once again, your body is confronted with changes in hormone levels.

And once again, your body must gradually get used to that. We can't say how long it takes because it varies for each woman and individual situation. Neither is there a correlation between how quickly you recovered from a previous pregnancy and how you will this time. The good news is that you have a major impact on that recovery process. You have the chance to be nice to your hormones before they become unbalanced.

## TRAINING TIPS

You can do these things to regain your hormone balance:

**1. Reduce stress.** Well, it's easier said than done when you only get a few hours' sleep a night, your whole life is upside down, and you have all new feelings. There's not much you can do about these factors right now.

But, of course, there are some factors that contribute to stress that you can do something about (e.g., how high you set the bar for yourself and where your priorities lie).

Stress has a more of a direct impact on your hormone levels than you might think. In your body, you have receptors that hormones can attach to. Only a bound hormone can do its job. Both the hormone progesterone (good for regaining the balance with estrogen in your body after childbirth) as well as the hormone cortisol (stress) fit on the same receptor. It's not a fair race, however; cortisol is much faster than progesterone. If you are incredibly stressed, all those cortisol hormones attach to the receptors, meaning progesterone has nowhere to attach itself. The major question is: what can and will you do about this? See it this way: every choice you make to do even a little something for yourself and to relax reduces your stress levels. Your body will get fewer signals to produce cortisol, which gives progesterone the chance to attach to a receptor and do its job properly.

So, you see, you don't have to throw all stress overboard to influence your cortisol levels because it is impossible to get rid of all stress, of course. But every little bit helps, and each time you decide to let it all go, you reduce the levels of stress hormones in your body and give progesterone a good chance to attach itself.

**2. Get rid of excessive weight!** Your fat cells can convert the counterpart of estrogen, testosterone, into estrogen. The more fat you have, the more estrogen you produce. You should lose weight sensibly of course, especially in this vulnerable period. Therefore, not from day one after the birth, but only once you are in the "To" phase. And even then, you should be careful when you are breast-feeding, for instance (see page 160).

## POSTPARTUM THYROIDITIS: INFLAMMATION OF THE THYROID

Hormones are also produced in the thyroid. The thyroid often starts working too fast in the year after childbirth, and this can cause countless "vague" symptoms, such as:

- An enlarged thyroid gland
- Nervousness, fear, feeling uptight or depressed, impatience, irritability
- Heart palpitations
- From flushing to excessive sweating
- Digestive issues
- Tiredness

A woman who has just had a baby could have any of these symptoms. Who isn't tired? Who doesn't have mood swings sometimes? Isn't forgetfulness part of life when so much has changed? The symptoms are actually so vague that the possibility of an enlarged thyroid gland is often overlooked. If you recognize these symptoms, ask your physician to examine your thyroid. You could be given treatment for depression while you are actually suffering from an inflammation of your thyroid gland.

And to make it even more complicated, after a period of the thyroid gland working too quickly, it can start working slowly for a while. Symptoms of an underactive thyroid gland (hypothyroidism) are:

- Enlarged thyroid gland
- Cold intolerance
- Weight gain but reduced appetite
- Tiredness, trouble concentrating, forgetfulness
- Constipation
- Proximal muscle weakness (muscle weakness and stiffness in the upper legs and arms, in particular)
- Feelings of depression
- Dry and pale skin
- Shortness of breath with exertion
- Reduction in the amount of breast milk

These symptoms are also hard to recognize, and once again: if you recognize a few of them, get your thyroid tested!

# YOU AND
# YOUR MIND

B esides all the physical changes, there is perhaps one change that tops them all: the changes in your mind—those things we can't put on an anatomical chart but that actually change the most.

# Back to You or a New You?

There is no doubting that you change when you become a mother. There is also no doubting that you are the same person and always will be. There is also no doubting how strange that might sound. But it's all true.

On the one hand, you are you and will always be you. You like certain things, have unique character traits, individual talents, and personal points for improvement. On the other, it's perfectly normal for you to notice changes in yourself now that you are a mother. Things that were irrelevant before you gave birth are suddenly very important to you. Things you liked before are boring now. Movies that did nothing for you, now make you cry.

To start with, it's incredibly important to accept this. Accept that your world has changed and that this can cause some insecurities and a search for "You." It's important that you seize this opportunity to make the right choices for your baby, for you right now and later, and for any relationship you have.

# The Changes in You

Every woman is unique and every woman changes, or experiences changes, in her own way. And yet, you will see that many women go through a number of similar changes. The difference is often in how consciously you deal with them.

### Change 1: Increased Sensitivity

Almost every woman experiences things more intensely and becomes more sensitive to stimuli from her surroundings after childbirth. On the one hand, it makes perfect sense due to—here they are again—the hormones. On the other, the structure of the brain has also changed, which makes you more empathic. This may serve a biological purpose, but these feelings can seem intense—sometimes so intense that even the strongest woman can suddenly start doubting everything or cry about the slightest thing. Almost every new mother becomes more sensitive. The wonderful emotions get even more wonderful, but the doubts can also hit you harder.

It helps if you are aware of the fact your feelings have changed. What things do you experience differently? Do you know why? How do these new emotions feel? Can you learn something positive from them or turn them into something positive? And however cliché it sounds, talk about it. Express how you feel and talk about the changes you are experiencing. If you tell those closest to you, they will understand you better. And when you feel understood, you feel better, which will help you give this new sensitivity a place in your life.

## Change 2: Reconsidering Norms and Values

A less well-known change but one experienced by many new mothers and fathers is different norms and values. You suddenly think differently about things. You want to make a different contribution to the world. Or perhaps you start thinking about it for the first time. You reconsider your role in society, regarding the environment, child labor, or social goals, for example. You start driving more responsibly, and you wait for the green light before crossing an empty road.

You are now responsible for a new generation, which makes you look at things in a new light. See it as a wonderful opportunity to reflect and see what you stand for. You might discover an even nicer side to yourself!

## Change 3: Forgetting Yourself

Brush your hair? Shower? Time to go to the bathroom in peace? And a pair of pants covered in stains is still a pair of pants, right? Your personal care can really suffer when you become a mother. You do everything for your baby, who looks tip-top, but you totally forget yourself. It's understandable, but you will need to find the balance again. You don't want to look in the mirror a few years down the line and think, "Well, there's nothing left of me. I work my fingers to the bone for everyone else, but where am I?"

## Change 4: New Job?

You loved your job, it was the most important thing to you, you always gave it your all, and then . . . you became a mother. Suddenly, your job is no longer the number one priority it used to be. Many women feel less career driven all of a sudden and want to enjoy this baby time to the fullest. This time passes so quickly. Your baby needs you and, indeed, children are big before you know it. That is why it's important to really think about your career and what you want in the long term. There are no wrong choices when you follow your feelings and heart and are realistic. Really think about your future and how the choices you make today will affect it.

## DR. SHEILA DE LIZ, gynecologist, Wiesbaden, Germany

Becoming a mother is an extremely intense experience, and it places great demands on your body and mind. See it as a chance to rediscover your internal super strength. Don't forget to think about yourself. Don't make choices that you will regret or blame others for later on. Think about who you are as a mother, what you stand for, whether you want to be/stay financially independent, and about the example you want to set for your children. When writing my book on menopause, I found that many women regret the choices they made when they became a mother. No matter how much they enjoyed motherhood, in hindsight they blamed themselves and their partner for a lack of space for themselves, feeling that they "served" the family all the time and that they couldn't continue their career the way they wanted to. Those types of things are difficult to change after the fact. This often results in women ending up in a relationship crisis or having issues with their self-image. I always encourage my clients to really think about their major life choices and not to forget themselves when doing that. Remember, you will feel better about yourself when you exercise, eat healthily, and look good. And you will radiate that—it's what you give off, and it makes you a lovely person, for yourself, your baby, your partner, your friends, and your colleagues.

Some food for thought:
- A career break is often an obstacle for further development later down the line. It's not fair, but it's a fact.
- Do you want to be financially dependent (or more so) on your partner?
- How many hours do you and your partner want to continue working?
- How are you going to divide work and household tasks between you both?
- Will you regret it later if you stop your career now?
- What example do you want to set for your baby?

And as if that's not enough to think about, many women also face a quite different question. Do I still want to do my current job? It could be that the commercial position you held no longer seems relevant and you start looking for other challenges to suit your new view of the world. Because your norms and values have changed, that could affect the way you think about your job. The decisions you make about your position, your work, your working hours, and your career have a major impact on the course of your life. Give it serious thought and talk about it at home, with friends, and perhaps with your HR manager.

Listen to everyone's advice and then make the decision that suits the new "You."

## Change 5: Your Social Network Becomes Less Important

You can fill up 40 hours a day and yet there will only ever be 24 of them. You run after your own shadow and time catches up with you. It becomes quite easy to forget your social network and your friends. You'll message them tomorrow. Didn't manage that. We'll meet up next week. And guess what? Nothing has happened a month later. Almost everyone will recognize this, but no matter how normal it is, it's good for you to have a good old chat and laugh every so often. You have a whole lot to deal with, and you can't discuss absolutely everything with your partner. Talking, taking time to relax, and focusing on yourself is important for a person. It makes perfect sense that your social calendar isn't as full as it used to be. But it doesn't have to be completely empty, either. And if your social calendar fills up, make sure you plan things around your baby and take more time than usual to lay things out, pack, and get everything and everyone else ready. You will be able to really enjoy the time and won't be stressed.

## Change 6: Forgetting Your Relationship

As easy as it is to forget yourself, it's just as easy to forget your relationship. You are both busy with your new role as father or mother, and all your care and attention go to your baby and to finding a new daily rhythm.

Of course, you don't start going on all kinds of romantic dates from week one. No one expects that, and it would be a little strange. Those first weeks are about surviving. But what you must watch out for is that you don't create new habits during that survival time: a habit of taking your relationship for granted and not seeing each other as lovers but only as joint caregivers. In the "Back" phase, that phase of surviving, try to talk to each other about what you are going through. Don't only share the facts but also your feelings. Talk about the changes, about the differences in how you expected it to be and how it really is (and there will be differences!). This will allow you to maintain intense contact in the period of transition and growth. When the "To" phase starts, it will be time to plan more time together. And during the "You" phase, remember that "you" can also mean both of you ;-).

### Change 7: Setting the Bar Too High

And then there's another change that three in four women recognize in themselves: you expect to have suddenly changed from a woman into Wonder Woman and Superwoman all in one. You think you should be able to do everything and much more. You don't set the bar high but higher than high. Sound familiar? Of course, it's great that you want the best for your baby, but be realistic: there is no such thing as a perfect parent. Just the fact you are trying makes you perfect. See the funny side of the impossible hoops you are jumping through and laugh about them. Think about how you got yourself into that position. What was so important that it had to be done? And were those elements really that important?

By analyzing the situation, you will also realize that demanding the impossible of yourself simply won't work, and next time you'll set that bar a little lower. Or, put another way, be more realistic. Set your priorities, look at what's really important, and leave it at that. Only do what's really necessary—anything more is too much at the moment and will only wear you down.

### Change 8: Doubting Yourself More Than Ever

Everyone knows that doubts get you nowhere. Although all those doubts could be a good thing, as they make you a better mother. When you doubt, you question whether you are acting in your baby's best interests. And that shows that you want to be the best you can for your baby. Doubting, therefore, does have a function. But if your doubts become so overwhelming that they affect your mindset, then they stop working in your favor. Before they change into a major influence on you, it's advisable to discuss those concrete doubts with someone close to you. Talk about them with a woman who is also a mother. You'll notice that everyone has had the same types of doubts. When you have had a baby before, you will be better able to recognize these feelings. But that doesn't offer any guarantees, either. Sometimes that "doubteritis" hits harder than with a previous baby. That's perfectly normal, too.

With all these changes, one thing's for sure: they are a process to get "Back To (a renewed) You." And remember, *sometimes you need to change to get closer to yourself.*

## From (Normal) Stress to Depression

You could notice some extreme changes in yourself. Or those around you think they are extreme. Doubting yourself is fairly normal, but doubting yourself too much is not good for you. It's normal to be anxious about doing something wrong, but if those fears take over your life, then it's time to tackle the situation. It's perfectly normal for you to ask yourself every so often why you ever thought it was a good idea to have children, but if it stops you from forming a bond with your baby, you need to get help. When you work on your own mental stability, it is not just for you but also for your baby.

First this: don't be embarrassed if you notice that, mentally, things aren't working as smoothly as before. Almost half of women experience some type of mental issue (e.g., restlessness, irritation, panic attacks), and one in five women have a severe psychological disorder after childbirth. One in five women means it's not that rare. All you have to do is be honest with yourself, and if you think you are "not totally okay," do something about it as soon as possible. The quicker you act, the easier it is to resolve the issue.

## PROF. ADRIAAN HONIG, psychiatrist, Amsterdam, the Netherlands

Here are two effective ways to help you determine whether you need to seek professional help:

1. Talk to your partner, a good friend, or your parents and tell them how you feel and what you are worrying about. Ask them whether they notice any changes in you. If so, ask them how they experience these changes. They can help you because they know you best. They may not be a therapist, but they are your first line of support and perhaps, therefore, even better than a therapist at judging the changes in you. If you are doubting your ability as a good mother, ask them. You may be getting all concerned because you have set the bar too high. They will be able to reassure you because they will most probably think and see that you are an exceptionally good mother.

2. If, after step 1, you think you might have psychological issues, take the HADS test you can find online from many hospitals. This questionnaire is designed to help physicians recognize anxiety disorders and types of depression. You can also complete it yourself to get an initial idea as to whether you need professional help.

If you score seven or higher on the HADS list, that's a reason to get professional help. If you've been to a psychologist before, it's advisable to see them again. After all, they know you already.

## Your Psyche and Disorders

Basically, you can differentiate between these five forms of psychological disorders:

- Postpartum stress (something we all have, actually!)
- Postpartum anxiety
- Post-traumatic stress disorder (PTSD)
- Postpartum psychosis
- Postpartum depression

## BRAIN FACT: CARE AND STRESS OVERLAP

Did you know that the region in the brain responsible for motherly care for your baby overlaps with the areas that play a role in stress? When that region of your motherly care is activated, that stress region is automatically activated, too.

### Postpartum Stress

Stress not only has a function, but a life without some type of stress is simply unrealistic. As a new parent, you are faced with a peak in stress. We call this postpartum stress. So much changes in your life, and that is accompanied by worries, anxiety, and therefore stress.

There's nothing wrong with that as long as the stress doesn't go beyond this "normal" form. But you should be aware of the fact that you are currently in a stressful period so that you can prevent the stress from having a detrimental impact on your life.

Two scientists, Thomas Holmes and Richard Rahe, have drawn up a list of life events that are stressful for people. You won't be surprised to hear that having a baby and all the accompanying changes (renovating the nursery, change of job, new financial position, etc.) score very highly on the stress list. Do the self-test on page 259 to get an idea of the life events and the degree to which they contribute to stress in your life.

This self-test is not meant to scare the life out of you. On the contrary, we just want to show you that:

- What you are going through, doing, and managing is no mean feat.
- It's perfectly normal for you to be stressed by it sometimes.
- Everyone who has a baby has a tough time every so often. Every pink cloud has gray flecks.
- You deserve to treat yourself every so often and take time for yourself.

## Postpartum Anxiety

Normal anxieties and stress can take on a severe form to the point where anxiety can affect how you function. Your stress levels are already being tested to the limits, and you won't be surprised to hear that an estimated one in five women experience this. The crazy thing is that postpartum anxiety is rarely spoken about. It is also often hard to distinguish from the normal stress and worries parents have. Everyone worries that they might accidentally drop their baby at some point. How can you differentiate "normal" anxiety from postpartum anxiety? On top of that, there is no distinct line between "normal stress" and an excessive level of stress.

Characteristics of postpartum anxiety are:

- You keep having recurring anxious thoughts. They seem to take over your mind to a certain degree.
- You could have panic attacks. You are suddenly overcome with extreme fear and panic, and it takes over your mind and body.
- You could feel restless, irritated, and rushed the whole time.
- You could feel it physically: pressure on your chest or very tense muscles.

**WARNING:** If you recognize any of these types of overwhelming anxieties in yourself and your head is all messed up, you need to get help: for you, your baby, and any partner you may have. The sooner you do that, the easier it will be to get those thoughts out of your head. The longer you carry them around, the more you will find yourself in a downward spiral. Talk to your friends or your family. Go to your family physician and ask them for advice. Talking anonymously in online groups can also be of help. Find the help you need, don't be embarrassed, and pay extra attention to factors that could help you rebalance your hormone levels (see page 57). In short, be aware of your diet, your rest, and your physical exercise. The mind tips in the BTY program will help you stay in control of stress and help you take that time for yourself (which also means doing good by your family).

## Post-Traumatic Stress Disorder (PTSD)

Until recently, it was thought that PTSD was a trauma people got from a traffic accident, a natural disaster, or war. We have since learned that you can also get PTSD from childbirth, especially if things didn't go as you imagined or your baby was in (life-threatening) danger. But it could also be caused by things such as the feeling of having to cope alone, a lack of support from your partner, the feeling that you are losing control, or a very painful, exceptionally long, or even very quick labor. In an ideal health-care system, the physician would do a basic check after labor to see whether a trauma has arisen during childbirth. PTSD can be treated by talking with a health professional. And if you think: people have been giving birth since time immemorial, so how come I am too weak to do it? Stop right there. That's where you are going wrong. Although very few women talk about it, it is more common than you might think. It's estimated that one in ten women have a birth trauma. Don't be embarrassed. Do something about it before the consequences of PTSD become more severe and you start to develop symptoms, such as depression.

## Postpartum Psychosis

Postpartum psychosis is characterized by irrational thoughts, seeing and hearing things that aren't there, hallucinating, or delusions and, even worse, a woman feeling that she wants to end her or her baby's life. If you have even the slightest concern that you could be experiencing psychosis or if those around you are questioning what you are saying, talk to your midwife or family physician immediately. Fortunately, postpartum psychosis can be successfully treated.

## Postpartum Depression

You could compare postpartum depression with the kinds of depression you could experience at any phase of your life. Anxiety or worries and negative thoughts don't just pop up occasionally; they don't seem to go away. Characteristics include:

- Despondent moods
- Bouts of crying
- Feeling empty or dead inside
- No interest in your baby or even disliking them
- Edginess, irritation, feelings of aggression
- Worrying
- Little self-confidence, feeling of powerlessness

It can be hard to tell the difference between post-traumatic stress disorder caused by childbirth and postpartum depression. In both cases it can be difficult to build a good bond with your baby. With PTSD, your mind is taken over by thoughts of the traumatic labor. Because you are constantly thinking about it, you are unable to enjoy your baby and build that bond.

With postpartum depression, you don't feel comfortable in your own skin and you can't enjoy your baby. There could be a direct cause for postpartum depression, at other times there isn't.

Several factors can contribute to experiencing postpartum depression. They are:

- **Biological factors:** Here they are again: the changing hormone levels, that are out of balance, a disrupted thyroid gland, a low glucose level, or a deficiency in some vitamins or minerals, such as $B_6$, $B_{12}$, iron, or zinc.
- **Psychosocial causes:** Consider the changes within you and your social network: the pressure on your relationship when you've just become a parent, any change in job, a renovation you have fit in, and all that combined with less sleep, a crying baby, and a changed you.
- **Psychological factors:** By this we mean, for example, all the changes described at the beginning of this chapter. You have set the bar too high, have not set your priorities in the best way for you, are not considering yourself enough, etc.
- **Genetic factors:** Recent studies show (once again) that there is a major link between nutrition, rest, exercise, and postpartum depression. We can't prevent all types of postpartum depression, but with the current knowledge, we can limit the effects as far as possible and even avert some types of depression. The Back To You program is a great help in that. You learn how your diet affects your hormones, we give you information about the importance of rest, and we give you the chance to create your own personal training schedule, all of which will result in you producing more positive substances in your body. The program also includes many practical and simple tips that will help you stay in control of stress.

## CRYING DURING THOSE FIRST DAYS

The baby blues are a well-known, worldwide phenomenon. Many women know exactly how the baby blues feel, but they have never been scientifically proven. This is a brief period, from a few hours to a few days, of feeling "down" or crying for no apparent reason. Baby blues are not comparable with genuine postpartum depression.

# THE XL
# FUNDAMENTALS

O kay, enough theory. Now you know all about the functions, the importance, and the effect of your pregnancy and parenthood on your brain, your powerhouse, your hormones, and your vagina. Now, for the practical part: how are you going to get all those elements into perfect shape? What do you need to do to feel comfortable in your own skin and mind, to heal your physical injuries, and to feel completely yourself again?

The XL Fundamentals are the key ingredients to become a better version of yourself.

They are game changers for now and for later, for you and your baby.

## The XL Fundamentals: For a Real Impact on You

These XL Fundamentals are the basis for a good recovery and a healthy lifestyle:

- Nutrition
- Rest and Relaxation
- Posture and Breathing
- Exercise and Training

And now for the amazing thing: you can tackle them individually and see results. When you start eating more healthily, your health will naturally improve. And that applies to all the fundamentals. But there's another remarkable thing about them. When you make all these key elements a fundamental part of your lifestyle, you increase the effect: 1 + 1 + 1 + 1 doesn't equal 4 but more like 8. When you combine them, you double the impact and they have an XL (extra-large) impact. There's a good reason we call them the *XL Fundamentals*.

# That Means a Lot of Changes . . .
# Nope. It Doesn't.

Don't be alarmed—it's easier than it seems and will even gain you some time!
You get more energy and can cope with more. In the following chapters, you
can read all about the XL impact of each individual fundamental and how it
influences the other fundamentals. In addition, we give you simple life hacks
to achieve major effects through small adjustments.

> Your weekly BTY program takes all the XL Fundamentals into
> account so that you see permanent change and to show you how
> easy it is to feel good and healthy in your body and mind.

# XL
# FUNDAMENTAL:
# NUTRITION

You could write a whole book about nutrition and the impact it has on your body and hormones. But that's probably one of the last things you want to focus on right now. For nine months, there were certain things you could and couldn't eat, and now that that's behind you, you have to think about your diet again! That's why we keep it simple here and only list a few tips that can have a real impact on your recovery. And they will also be valuable for the rest of your life.

# 10 Golden Nutrition Tips

Here they are, the 10 ways to adjust your diet. They are not 10 commandments, and you are allowed to sin as well. Just try to apply the tips as often as possible, without feeling like you have to change a whole lot or give up many things. You'll notice it's fairly easy and will get even easier.

1. Eat "honest" foods.
2. Choose organic and unpackaged foods.
3. Avoid sugar and refined carbohydrates.
4. Avoid foods your body has an adverse reaction to.
5. Eat vegetables. Lots and lots and lots.
6. Add nuts and seeds.
7. Eat fiber-rich foods.
8. Limit alcohol, coffee, smoking, and even nonprescription medication.
9. Consider taking nutritional supplements.
10. Beware of unintentional "foods."

## 1. "Honest" Products

A pineapple that is a pineapple, a tomato that is a tomato. That is honest food. As soon as the pineapple is canned or juiced in a factory, it's not a pineapple anymore. The same applies to a tomato that is no longer a tomato after it has been pureed or skinned and canned. Healthy substances are lost when products are processed, and those substances are extremely healthy for your body. Buying whole, honest products and preparing them yourself gives you energy.

And, by doing this, you will also make the best breast milk, the healthiest, honest first food for your baby. And another plus: your baby's microbiome (the gut bacteria population) will be extremely healthy, which is good for the immune system and means your child will be sick less often. Honest food is also honest for your body.

## 2. Choose Organic and Unpackaged as Far as Possible

All groceries that aren't organic have been treated with agricultural toxins to encourage growth or make them less vulnerable. This provides the highest possible profits from these products. You pay less money for these products than for the organic varieties, but your body pays a higher price. These products often disrupt your hormonal balance, and their nutritional value is generally lower. And that's not all. The plastic packaging doesn't improve things, either, to put it lightly. It releases hazardous substances, of which we can't even oversee the consequences. Recent studies have shown that we have drastically underestimated the effects until now. Therefore, eating organic and unpackaged food as much as possible is really the best choice for your body and your baby. (See also phytoestrogens, page 82.)

## 3. Avoid Sugar (Substitutes) and Refined Carbohydrates

You could almost say that sugar is one of the most popular drugs. It gives you an instant kick, and, in fact, heavily processed products with sugar are even addictive. And then we are talking about refined sugar, which is added to sodas (six cubes a glass!) and found in candy and cookies. And, less well known, sugar is also added to mayonnaise (!), processed meats such as hot dogs, and fruit yogurts and breakfast drinks.

Each time you ingest lots of sugar, you experience that "kick." But your body will also produce vast amounts of insulin to stabilize your blood sugar-level. Once that "kick" has passed, your body is left with that blood sugar-lowering insulin. The result: you feel drowsy and look for more energy, which you find in the form of sugar. That gives you another kick, followed by a sugar dip, followed by a craving, etc. And it only gets worse each time.

There are natural sugars in almost all our plant-based foods, from the obvious fruit (fruit sugars) to grains. But nature has a clever trick up her sleeve: each item of food, whether an apple or grain of rice, also contains exactly the right amount of nutritional fiber. That perfect balance means you don't consume excessive amounts of sugar because the nutritional fiber inhibits the absorption of sugars in the blood.

It's a different matter, though, when you disrupt Mother Nature's perfect balance by removing a specific part of the food: consider pressed apple juice, white rice, white bread, pasta, etc. All these refined products ensure a relatively high sugar absorption and, therefore, an increase in the blood sugar level, meaning your body starts producing more insulin.

And what's the deal with those natural sweeteners, such as high-fructose syrups? They are often nothing more than a big marketing trick. Yes, it's a natural fruit sugar, but in a processed and highly concentrated form. High-fructose syrup is one of the reasons that people unintentionally gain weight or that they are unable to lose weight.

Therefore, check the label before buying something that supposedly contains only natural products.

A high insulin level disrupts a woman's normal menstrual cycle. It's vital to regain that cycle after pregnancy. And that's what the body struggles with and what it starts doing right after the placenta has left the womb. Your body wants to return to a cycle, and added sugars and refined carbohydrates work against that.

## 4. Avoid Food Your Body Has an Adverse Reaction To

Your body often lets you know what it does and doesn't react well to. We are not talking about a food intolerance or allergy, but foods that just don't agree with you. They make you feel bloated or give you a visibly swollen belly, for instance. It doesn't mean you are allergic or intolerant, but those foods are not good for you. When you eat those products too often, your immune system goes into overdrive and your body becomes stressed. When you are stressed, your body produces excessive levels of stress hormones and they, in turn, disrupt the natural cycle. Your body alone can tell you what it reacts to, but gluten, lactose (milk protein), and casein (milk sugar) are known for the adverse effect they have on a large number of people. We are increasingly finding that people can't cope with these things and they feel better when they decrease the amounts they consume. Avoid these products if you notice your body has an adverse reaction to them.

### DR. JOLENE BRIGHTEN, naturopathic physician, biochemist, and female hormone expert, Seattle, USA

After the delivery, your body could suddenly react badly to different things, and your body may suddenly be able to tolerate certain things it couldn't cope with before. Pregnancy also disrupts your food sensitivities and intolerances. Try it out. If you notice your body suddenly reacts badly to something, don't consume it for about six months. After those six months, you could give it another go, and your body may well be able to handle it again. Also check if your former sensitivities and intolerances are still there. If you keep having issues, see your physician.

# 5. Eat Vegetables. Lots and Lots of Vegetables.

The standard is 10.5 ounces of vegetables a day. And although that may be enough to get your daily vitamins and minerals, it's not enough for your diet to contribute to your recovery. Your body can only perform miracles to the max when you eat 17.6 ounces of vegetables per day. That sounds impossible, and if you only eat vegetables with your evening meal, it will be. Therefore, eat vegetables with every meal. Even with breakfast, even as a snack. We are not talking about eating green beans for breakfast but perhaps some slaw or a healthy smoothie. Or toss some vegetables in a wok and put them in an omelet. Don't put a sweet topping on your cracker but a slice of avocado instead. Or make baba ghanoush, a lovely smooth spread made with grilled eggplant. Hummus, made with chickpeas, is also an easy and healthy spread. Have a salad or soup for lunch more often. It doesn't take long to make soup: make a big pan in one go and it'll last a few days. You can also have a cup of soup as a snack during the day. Easy does it. See it this way: every bite of vegetables you take before your evening meal is a bonus.

## TIP: PUT CABBAGE ON THE MENU

One vegetable deserves special attention: cabbage. A substance called diindolylmethane (DIM) grows in, or should we say on, cabbage. This substance helps reduce the dominance of estrogens in your body. DIM is on cabbage anyway but grows even more where the cabbage is "broken." If you cut or bruise the cabbage and put the cut and bruised vegetable to the side for a while before preparing and eating it, even more DIM grows on the cabbage. Almost all types of kimchi contain a lot of cabbage, too, and due to the fermentation process they also contain lots of probiotic bacteria (particularly good for your immune system), and fermentation removes specific substances from the cabbage that are potentially not as good for your body. Another benefit of kimchi or other fermented vegetables is that they have a long shelf life and can be added to your lunch as an extra to turn it into a three-in-one health bomb: therefore, you get vegetables, probiotics, and DIM in a few bites. The combination of eating cabbage and breastfeeding can cause some babies to get more cramps, though. Keep this is mind if you are breastfeeding. However, you don't have to avoid cabbage from the outset.

## 6. Add Nuts and Seeds

Nuts are filled with good substances. Each type of nut has something special about it. Hazelnuts contain lots of vitamin E, macadamia nuts contain a lot of zinc, and walnuts and split flaxseeds are a plant-based source of omega-3 fatty acids, which are good for the brain. Sunflower seeds contain massive amounts of iron, zinc, and magnesium. And how about chestnuts? They score high in folic acid.

But watch out: we are talking about raw nuts here and not roasted or salted nuts that could have lost nutrients through processing methods.

Peanuts have a relatively low nutritional value and contain a lot of fat. Interesting fact: almonds are officially fruit and peanuts are legumes. As they have a similar nutritional value to nuts, they are often mentioned in the same breath.

Seeds are filled to the brim with all kinds of healthy elements, such as minerals, vitamins, and antioxidants. They also have another major benefit: they can easily be added to almost anything you eat. Sprinkle them through a salad, over your soup, or on your sandwich.

## 7. Eat Fiber-Rich Foods

Vegetables (yes, here they are again), whole-grain products, and nuts contain fiber. There are two types of fiber: fermentable and nonfermentable. The fermentable fiber is broken down by the bacteria residing in the bowels. Part of that fermentable fiber is also meant to provide the gut flora with food. These are so-called prebiotics: goodies for your gut microbiome (see page 85).

The second type, the nonfermentable fiber, can't be broken down in the body. But it still has an important task. It helps prevent constipation (hard stools) because it holds on to a lot of fluid, which makes pooping easier. Constipation is not good for your pelvic floor. It makes you push more often, and your pelvic floor doesn't want to undergo that pushing (every day). It cramps your muscles and puts a massive amount of pressure on a region that, in fact, needs to relax.

Fun fact: vegetables that grow above ground have more fiber, and vegetables that grow below ground contain more starch.

## 8. Limit Alcohol, Coffee, Smoking, and Even Nonprescription Medication

All these substances disrupt your natural hormone balance. And you need balanced hormones to prevent yourself from getting countless health issues (postpartum, but also for the rest of your life). Obviously, you should not stop taking any prescription medication, but do think twice before taking over-the-counter drugs.

Pain also has a function: it warns you when you are demanding too much of your body. And your body is often a very good adviser!

## 9. Consider Taking Nutritional Supplements

Some nutrients are lacking in our food. That means it is becoming increasingly difficult to ingest enough B vitamins, for example. $B_{12}$ is mainly found in animal products. Animals don't make them themselves, the bacteria in their intestinal tract do. Many experts believe that animals themselves have a $B_{12}$ deficiency nowadays because the composition of their gut flora has changed over time. We have changed the way we treat animals and what we feed them, and that influences their gut microbiome. That could explain why animals' meat, milk, or eggs lack $B_{12}$ nowadays.

It's important to take extra $D_3$, especially in the months when there is less sunlight. It is not found in food; you get it from the sun.

You could consider taking D-mannose for your bladder (unless you are breastfeeding) and magnesium for your pelvic floor and other muscles (see page 29). A daily dose of vitamin C-1000 can do wonders for your immune system.

## 10. Be Careful with Unintentional "Foods"

We also ingest things that are not food. These are things like that last bit of toothpaste, your lip balm, microscopic particles of food packaging, Teflon flakes from a damaged pan, etc.

## YOUR BODY AND MIND: UNDER THE INFLUENCE OF YOUR GUT FLORA

We used to believe that the intestines were little more than the tube your stools came out of. That's the biggest underestimation ever. The intestinal wall contains our so-called second brain. That second brain can communicate with the central nervous system, but it can also work independently. Billions of bacteria, and about 150 different types, live in the intestines. The composition of these bacteria is largely responsible for whether your body is healthy or not. If your gut microbiome (gut flora population) is healthy, then it can combat disease for you through your immune system and you will feel energetic, strong, and good. If your gut microbiome is disrupted, you will get sick quicker, it will take longer to recover (also after the delivery!), and you will feel weaker and less comfortable in your own skin. In fact, recent studies not only show a direct link between your gut microbiome and your immune system but also a direct link between postpartum depression and the gut microbiome. Other mental illnesses and incontinence can also be linked to a poorly functioning gut microbiome. And how does that gut microbiome develop? It comes from the food and other substances we ingest.

The intestines and gut microbiome also play a vital role in breaking down estrogens. A disrupted gut flora population can cause certain estrogens to split, and they are transported back into the body rather than being excreted.

In short, a healthy diet is essential, and it plays a vital role in preventing and improving numerous symptoms you could experience after childbirth.

## DR. JOLENE BRIGHTEN, naturopathic physician, biochemist, and female hormone expert, Seattle, USA

Research has shown that trauma to the head, for example, has a direct influence on your gut microbiome. The content of the gut flora population is replaced within 72 hours of a head trauma. There haven't been any studies into the effect of the physical trauma on the intestines after childbirth, but it does get you thinking. If the physical trauma of childbirth also affects our digestive system, we should take better care of our intestines after having a baby.

These are all things we consume through our mouths but that are not real food, and we are not aware we are doing it.

Your mouth is not the only organ that consumes. Your skin also "eats" in a certain way. It is your largest organ, and it forms a barrier between your body and the outside world, but that barrier is not completely sealed. Most products that come into contact with the skin don't penetrate farther than the cornified layer, and they can do no harm there. It is a layer consisting of accumulated dead skin cells that creates a kind of wall around the rest of your body. But some substances can get through that cornified layer. Recent studies show that certain suntan lotions can enter the bloodstream, as can some drugs (medicinal salves or creams) and some over-the-counter pain-relieving creams or gels, for example.

And consider the chemicals in some tampons. Let's do the math: when you have your period every month and bleed for five days each time and use tampons, then you use $12 \times 5 = 60$ days (two full months!) of tampons per year. That is one-sixth of a year. So, as you can see, your blood isn't only fed by things you eat but also by things you unwittingly ingest.

The fact that you unwittingly ingest more things than desired also affects your hormone levels. Take estrogen, for example. Besides our body's own estrogens, there are two other types of estrogen-like substances that we ingest:

- **Phytoestrogens** (plant-based estrogens) can be found in almost all plant-based products, but in extremely high levels in soy, soy products, and hops.
- **Xenoestrogens** (from plastic, cosmetics, preservatives, and pesticides) are strong; no, they are extremely strong. They are many times stronger than our body's own estrogens and the plant-based estrogens. You could say that they are too strong for our body and so you should avoid them if you can. Xenoestrogens have a massive impact on your hormones. Therefore, it is even more important for you to avoid these extremely strong estrogens when your body is in a phase where it's having trouble with hormones anyway, whether that is while you are recovering from childbirth or later during menopause. Xenoestrogens are not only in food but also in other products we ingest through the mouth, such as plasticizers, pesticides, and preservatives. Plasticizers are hidden in your food when they are released from plastic packaging, a drink carton, or a can, for instance.

In short, if you choose pure, organic, and unpackaged products, you prevent any extra estrogens from sneaking into your body.

## TRAINING TIPS

- **Don't underestimate the role of nutrition.** Nutrition, combined with rest and training, determine how we feel, physically and mentally.
- **Consider substituting milk products with plant-based varieties** if your body reacts adversely to milk products. You could try oat milk or coconut yogurt.
- **Many meat substitutes contain soy, but not all.** A lot of soy has high levels of genetically modified organisms (GMO), and you want to avoid that. Pick a non-GMO organic variety. Check the label.
- **Listen to your body:** it is the best at telling you what it reacts well to.
- **Avoid monosodium glutamate.** This culprit is also known under the names MSG, glutamate, glutamic acid, hydrolyzed vegetable protein, gelatin, vetsin, potassium and sodium caseinate, added yeast, yeast extract, and monopotassium glutamate.

Monosodium glutamate is used as a flavor enhancer, making your food so tasty that you overeat. It stops your brakes, you could say. You keep eating, your stomach is full; you unzip your pants and yet still pile on another plateful. It stops you from listening to your body. And monosodium glutamate does even more, ranging from a bloated feeling or muscle aches to feeling weak, breathing difficulties, diarrhea—the list of possible symptoms caused by monosodium glutamate could go on and on. And because this list is so long and varied, it is extremely easy to confuse a typical postpartum health issue with a reaction to monosodium glutamate.

# PRE- AND PROBIOTICS: MIRACLE WORKERS FOR YOUR GUT MICROBIOME

You can help your gut microbiome by taking prebiotics and probiotics. But what is the difference between them and where do you find them?

## PROBIOTICS

Probiotics are good bacteria for your gut microbiome. Even your gut microbiome changed during your pregnancy. Mother Nature has ensured that it has become simpler, consisting of fewer distinct types of bacteria. We don't know why that is, but we do know that you need to regain a more complex microbiome filled with all the different bacteria. Therefore, it's time to get those good bacteria inside you again. You can take them as supplements, but you can also get them from natural products. These are often products that have been processed in a natural way, for example through fermentation. Try to eat the following products regularly:

1. **Yogurt:** During the fermentation process, the lactose is converted into lactic acid by lactic bacteria. This means yogurt is easy to digest and the probiotic bacteria do wonders for your intestines.

2. **Miso:** If you've not heard of this before, it's time to give it a go. Miso is a type of condiment paste you can use in sauces, or you can make a cup of souplike stock with it. It is made from fermented soybeans and a good miso soup can contain over 150 distinct types of bacteria. Not only that, but it is also low in calories and rich in B vitamins and antioxidants.

3. **Sauerkraut:** When cabbage is fermented, it creates good substances for your intestines. A daily dessert spoon of sauerkraut is particularly good for you. Try it as a snack or put it in a sandwich much like you would slaw. Sauerkraut is also filled with vitamin C.

4. **Pickles:** Pickles can be fantastic for your gut flora, too. Choose salted pickles prepared without vinegar. They might take a bit of getting used to, but they are very tasty in slices on a sandwich or as a snack during the day.

5. **Kefir:** It's relatively new on our Western menu, but the product is ancient, in fact. Kefir is made by adding kefir grains to milk. The milk ferments and you get a carbonated drink filled with

probiotics. You can buy ready-made kefir, but read the label. Many long-life kefir products contain few probiotics but many additives that are not good for you.

## PREBIOTICS

Prebiotics are food ingredients for the good bacteria in the intestines; they encourage the growth of these good bacteria. You can find them in many vegetables, fruit, whole-grain bread, grain products, and legumes. You can also take probiotics as a supplement.

Following are the four most well-known types of prebiotics and the products you can find them in:

1. **Inulin** is in the roots of plants that grow in moderately cold regions. Examples are salsify, Jerusalem artichoke, chicory, leek, and artichokes.
2. **Fructo-oligosaccharides (FOS)** can be found in bananas, asparagus, onion, and garlic.
3. **Galacto-oligosaccharides (GOS)** are in legumes, beans, cashew nuts and pistachio nuts, beets, broccoli, barley, and (oat) bran.
4. **Pectin** can be found in fruit—red currants, blackberries, lemons, plums, and oranges in particular.

**Fun Fact:** Breast milk can contain 130 types of oligosaccharides! There are hardly any in cow's milk.

# XL
# FUNDAMENTAL: REST AND RELAXATION

**J**ust as your pelvic floor muscles need to relearn to function in the full range of motion, so does your mind. You can only get the most energy out of life when you can also rest completely. There are actually two types of rest, namely sleep and mental relaxation. Both contribute to your recovery and to a better life.

## I WANT TO SLEEP AND RELAX BUT . . . HOW AND WHEN CAN I?!

You are not the only mother who really wants to sleep and relax but simply doesn't get the chance. However, there are methods you can use to make it easier to get some sleep and take time to rest without giving your number one priority, your baby, less attention or love. The exercises and tips in your BTY program help you with that. When you understand the XL impact of rest and relaxation, you might put them higher up on your list of priorities. First, let's look at some theory before we put it into practice.

# Sleep

Stress negatively affects your hormone balance because stress inhibits other hormones from doing their jobs properly. Sleep and rest have a positive effect on your testosterone and human growth hormone (HGH) levels and can decrease stress. And sleep and rest are the things that aren't easy to get when you have a baby. Those uninterrupted eight hours of sleep are probably a thing of the past. Instead of getting yourself all wound up looking for your baby's magical, nonexistent "sleep button," there are things you can adjust so that your body gets the rest it deserves.

## The Importance of a Natural Day-Night Rhythm

Our body is naturally programmed to enter a night rhythm when it gets dark and a day rhythm when it's light. That day-night rhythm influences our sleep-waking rhythm as well as all the associated rhythms; for instance, the amount of urine we produce (less at night than during the day) and our body temperature (lower at night, higher during the day). All those rhythms react to one another and are directed by hormones. In turn, the brain sends signals to those hormones when it does or doesn't perceive light. A great fact, but we no longer live in the way nature intended us to. When it gets dark, we turn on a light, which messes up our natural rhythm. Nowadays, it is, of course, impossible to live a life without lights and go to bed at 5 p.m. in winter, but there are other things we can do. Dim the lights in the evening and crawl under the blankets a little earlier in winter. You could also use a Himalayan salt lamp in the evening. It gives off a redder light, making it easier for your body to produce melatonin.

## The Effect of Screens on Your Sleep

Screens emit a very intense, bright blue light and radiation. These break down your melatonin. Therefore, put your cell phone in dark or night mode, or try to reduce your screen time in the hours before going to bed. Or, even better, ban screens altogether in the two hours before bed.

## LIGHT AND YOUR MENSTRUAL CYCLE

Just to emphasize how much light affects your body: it has been shown that light can influence a woman's ovulation and menstrual cycle.

### DR. JOLENE BRIGHTEN, naturopathic physician, biochemist, and female hormone expert, Seattle, USA

Don't switch on the light when baby wakes at night. Exposure to light, however short, affects your circadian rhythm. And not only yours, your baby's, too. Keeping it dark at night helps your baby get used to a day and night rhythm, and your child will learn to sleep at night quicker. It's not sleep training but a very natural way to guide your baby's physiological processes toward a good sleeping rhythm. Consider using a red lamp that you wear on your forehead. It will allow you to see where you are going but won't disrupt either of your circadian rhythms.

## The Effect of Power Naps

If you can't get a full night's sleep, you will need to grab a few extra hours during the day. Power naps are incredibly powerful and have proven to be effective for catching up on a lack of sleep. It is a misunderstanding that you catch up on a lack of sleep by sleeping longer the following night. Moreover, the chance that you can get an extra hour's sleep with a baby is as good as zero. NASA has shown that the best way to catch up on a lack of sleep is to have a 90-minute mini nap the following day for every hour of sleep you missed the night before. So, an hour and a half. You may be able to manage that, but you won't always be able to fit it into your schedule. In that case, have a genuine *power nap* of 20 minutes. That sounds like an extremely specific number, and there's a reason for that. If you sleep longer, you go into a deep sleep and you won't want to be rudely awakened from that. When you sleep only 20 minutes, your body and mind will have gotten a good rest, but you won't have fallen into a deep sleep.

## Take a Timeout Before Carrying On

When you have just become a mother, it's extremely easy to neglect your own rest. It makes perfect sense, considering there are a hundred things you have to do for your baby that are more important right now. Or . . . they seem more important. Looking after yourself and taking a break every so often is also a way of taking care of your baby. When you feel comfortable in your own skin, you can be a better mother. Those moments of rest don't have to cost you extra time if you are smart about how you tackle them. It's about regularly taking a few minutes for yourself and doing that very consciously. It's often that awareness that makes all the difference: take a moment for yourself and think about the amazing life you have. Give yourself these brief moments of reflection and of happiness.

## TRAINING TIPS

- **Some of the exercises are purely for your mind** (such as the relaxation exercises). They pep you up and promote your recovery because they have a positive effect on your hormone levels and your training results.
- **Ask yourself the questions:** What is the most important thing I should be doing when my baby naps during the day? Is that doing a chore or giving myself some rest so that I can better cope with the rest of the day? It may sound like a stupid question, but I see so many mothers who forget to think about themselves. *Back To You!* applies here, too. You really must go back to yourself every so often, forget that perfect picture, and grab some rest. You deserve it!
- **It is extremely good for you to see sunlight in the daytime.** It directly reduces your melatonin levels, making you feel more alert, more energetic, and happier. After all, melatonin is the hormone your body needs to feel tired. So, seeing a lot of light

is also good for your nightly sleep. The light makes your body produce more serotonin during the day, meaning you can produce more melatonin at night and you can get to sleep more easily. A third benefit is that the body produces vitamin D in sunlight, which we often already have a deficiency of outside the summer months.

- **An hour before going to sleep, read a book or do a meditation exercise.** That hour will give your body a chance to slow down and switch more smoothly from your day to night rhythm.

# Relaxation

Call it mindfulness or just chilling; call it a hobby or simply enjoying a moment, or call it doing nothing at all. One thing's for sure: it's important to let go and relax your mind to be able to exert it again.

## Pure Brain and Hormone Logic

Brain research has shown that if you don't get enough relaxation, the part of your brain that contributes to your memory, the hippocampus, suffers. You become more forgetful, which can be highly frustrating. Forgetting those silly little things you wouldn't normally forget is a typical signal of "too much tension." Parts of the frontal brain also suffer under too much stress. These regions contain your planning skills and your decision-making skills. So, here too: if you feel that you have lost sight of the overall picture, your schedule is all over the place, and you are indecisive, it's time for more relaxation.

On a hormonal level, relaxation instantly tackles all stress hormones. As soon as you relax, the happy hormones beat the stress hormones. Every second you relax, your body wins such a hormonal battle. Sitting down and drinking that cup of tea instead of guzzling it down while doing 101 other things does wonders for you. Your hormones react reasonably quickly, so you don't have to do hours of meditation or walking to get an effect. Those brief moments that you can easily adjust often have a significant impact. You won't get there with only brief moments, but they help immensely.

## Take a Moment to Think about the Things That Make You Happy

It's incredible, but as people, we tend to stop and think about the things that make us unhappy rather than those that make us happy. Other people give us more empathy and love when we share our problems than when we share our happy times. It's very, very strange because it's almost as if problems are rewarded, though research shows that stopping and thinking about positive things is much better for you. Therefore, get into a new habit of taking a moment to stop and think about what you are doing, about what you mean for your baby, the strength your body and mind had to create your little miracle. Enjoy the little things: the birds chirping as they announce the morning, your partner's lovely twinkling eyes, that delicious salad with your favorite nuts. Every day is filled with brief moments of happiness. Focus on them. Enjoy. Share your joy. Write them down. Dream about them.

Whatever you do: stop and think about the small things that, subconsciously, have an enormous impact and help your mind relax.

## Typical Mom-Can't-Relax Pitfalls

**NOT HAVING TIME:** Keep in mind that relaxation doesn't have to cost time. You can relax by living in the now, grabbing brief moments, and resetting yourself every so often by focusing on your breathing for a few minutes. Call it mindfulness or meditation, or simply just thinking about yourself for a moment. And you really can find a few minutes.

*You don't have to choose between being a good mom or thinking about yourself.* You really can do both. Setting priorities often fails with (if you take a moment to think about it) the insignificant things, such as making sure the house is in perfect order. With everything that costs time, ask yourself whether it really contributes to a better life. Is it really that important right now?

**AIMING FOR PERFECTION:** As soon as you have a baby, there's only one thing you want and that is to do everything perfectly. Actually, more perfect than perfect. You will be the best mother ever, and your child will only see the good side of you. Let's wake you up from that dream because you will never be perfect. And in fact, aiming for perfection will wear you down at a certain point and cause the exact opposite situation. By setting the bar too high for yourself, you will produce more stress hormones. Instead of aiming for perfection, try to show that you are doing your best. That's a wonderful life lesson to pass on to your child. The people who are open to learn in life are the happiest people.

**IT'S HARDER TO DO FUN THINGS SPONTANEOUSLY:** You might give yourself less time for relaxation now than you used to. It makes sense, really. It's simply impossible to spontaneously leave the house with your partner now. Accept that you will probably get out less in this period, you will have to plan more, and it's harder to do things spontaneously with a baby. After all, you must be at home on time because baby needs to nap, or you need to arrange a babysitter. But there is a difference between never doing anything fun and doing less. If you can't be spontaneous right now, then it's time to plan things instead and make sure you get out every so often without your baby.

NO TIME FOR A SOCIAL LIFE:  This pitfall is somewhat like that of having no time and setting priorities, but it's also particularly important to think about it. When your whole life has been turned upside down and time is catching up with you anyway, it's easy to unintentionally forget your social life. You see less of your friends, message them less, and at a certain point you may even think about them less. It's not because you don't care about them anymore but simply because parenthood can take some getting used to. And yet, it's important that you don't forget your social life. Hanging out with other people makes you a nicer person and you can be yourself for a while. You relax and recharge your batteries. Of course, your social calendar doesn't have to be as full as it was before baby, but it doesn't have to be empty, either.

## TRAINING TIP: A RESET DAY

You may have heard of them: reset days. If you've eaten fatty foods or too much one day, then you eat frugally and very healthily the next day. You balance the excesses of the one day with restraint the following day. You can also do the same with your mind. If you've had a busy day, take it easier the next day and get some rest.

# XL FUNDAMENTAL: POSTURE AND BREATHING

If there is one XL Fundamental that has a direct impact on the distribution of pressure in the abdominal cavity, it's your posture and breathing. Do you turn your feet inward when you walk? If so, that bad foot positioning puts the wrong pressure on your powerhouse, which, for example, could give you issues with your pelvic floor or back. Also, the way you lift an object affects the pressure you put on your pelvic floor. Your posture and your powerhouse influence your breathing, and your breathing affects the pressure on your powerhouse. It's actually fairly simple once you understand the principle behind it. The importance of posture and breathing is often underestimated. You can do training three times a week, but if you always put the wrong pressure on your powerhouse 24/7 because your posture and breathing are wrong, then those three training sessions really won't compensate for that.

> To make it simple and visualize it: imagine your powerhouse as a balloon sitting between your midriff, pelvic floor, and flanks. As soon as there is pressure on one of those spots, as if you are pinching one side of the balloon, there will be more pressure on the other side. And where will it go wrong? At the weakest spot. *Guess what*? That is often your pelvic floor or, if you have a hernia or large diastasis, it will be the spot of that hernia or diastasis. Good posture and breathing ensure that your balloon's weak spot doesn't come under extra pressure.

## Posture

Everything, and we mean everything, in your body starts with good posture. And no, we don't always naturally adopt the right posture with certain movements. You must teach yourself good posture. Do it and you will really be giving yourself a head start. Poor posture can harm your back, which affects other parts of your body. You will be trying to avoid the pain and will adopt another bad posture to compensate. You land in a vicious downward spiral.

Good posture ensures:

**OPTIMUM LEVELS OF OXYGEN:** If you don't have a straight posture (e.g., you are leaning forward or backward), you can't breathe optimally. You won't inhale a full dose of oxygen. You won't be aware of it, but you will definitely feel the difference once you get used to adopting a straight posture! Those extra few portions of oxygen are excellent for your muscles, your blood, your health, and your mind! When you lean forward while sitting or standing, your body must constantly work harder to get enough oxygen. Poor posture distorts the muscles, which restricts breathing because it is blocked somewhat.

**PROPER USE OF YOUR POWERHOUSE:** Your powerhouse provides by far the most stability and mobility when it is not crushed, lopsided, or bent. Bad posture can also negatively affect your pelvic floor muscles, one of the parts of your powerhouse. Poor posture can inhibit or slow down the recovery of slack or even cramped pelvic floor muscles; there is a higher risk of getting a prolapse or of its getting worse, and it is harder for a diastasis to recover.

**NO BAD STRAIN ON YOUR MUSCLES:** When you adopt a bad posture, you continually strain your muscles in the wrong way, which prevents them from resting. That can cause your muscles to cramp, which can weaken them. They don't get any rest due to being under constant tension.

**NO WRONG TYPE OF PRESSURE ON THE BONES:** Poor posture forces the bones to adopt an unnatural position. With every bad position, the bones come under pressure, they are compressed. Compression isn't always bad; in fact, compression on the bones is actually good when training. It only goes wrong when the compression is too frequent, lasts for too long, and is not targeted. For example, compare your vertebrae to an accordion that you can pull in and out. When you bend it, specific points move closer together or against each other. If you do it too often, too hard, or too long, the places where the points, or in this case your bones, touch each other will wear out.

**THE CORRECT TRAINING METHOD:** You can't train properly when you adopt a bad posture. Otherwise, you'll strain muscles that you shouldn't be straining. Or you won't be able to "reach" the right muscle group because your body posture is restricting the connection. It is therefore important to pay attention to your posture with every exercise. With every BTY exercise, you can read exactly what you should and, above all, should not do.

**A POWERFUL APPEARANCE:** When you walk and sit with a straight posture, you radiate self-confidence and energy. You'll notice it in the way others look at you, which will make you feel even better. You get into an upward spiral!

With a straight, proud posture, you will also feel stronger and prouder than with a weak, slouched posture. Try it out. Walk a little with a slouched posture and then walk straight and proud. Can you feel the difference?

**SMOOTHER TRIPS TO THE BATHROOM:** Or in plain English: with a good posture, you will be able to urinate and pass stools easier and better. It prevents unintentional damage to your anus, such as wounds, fissures, and even hemorrhoids. And it ensures that your pelvic floor muscles, which have already had a lot to endure, are not strained in the wrong way and become even more damaged in the process. Furthermore, a good toilet position helps you empty your bladder completely: to remove all urine in your urinary tract. If you don't empty your bladder completely, you could develop issues, such as a bladder infection (see page 103).

## IT SEEMS OVER THE TOP

Yes, everyone walks, stands still, sits down, and gets up throughout the day, and we've been doing that for decades. So, it seems a little over the top to have to learn that now. But that's not the case. Hardly anyone has perfect posture. Almost everyone quickly does that little thing, such as instead of bending your legs when you want to lift something, it's much quicker to bend your back. And who sits up nice and straight the entire day? Who really walks with their shoulders back, neck straight, and head straight ahead all day long? You can really score lots of points with good posture.

Here, you can read what all these ideal postures look like. And don't skip this part because you think it's over the top. It's vital and will give you lots and lots of benefits. So, you have just become a mother, yet you are going to relearn how to sit, stand, and lift. As you follow the weeks of training in the BTY program, you will notice that you start doing these types of things naturally.

## ALWAYS KEEP A LOOSE NECK

Whatever you do, whether you are sitting, lifting, turning, or standing up: make sure your neck is loose. Prevent tension in your neck. Don't get the strength from your neck but from other body parts, the parts you need to tighten for a specific movement. Your neck muscles should be loose and relaxed.

## Sitting

When you have just given birth (you are in the "Back" phase, 0–6 weeks, of your recovery), sitting could feel slightly strange and painful. But it's important that you sit upright and on a slightly hard surface. So, don't put a cushion under your butt, and instead sit on a chair that isn't too soft. That sounds painful, but it will really help and contribute to the recovery of your pelvic floor muscles. Listen to your body and don't do anything that really hurts. If you feel pain coming on, it's a signal to lie down. Don't try to compensate with a cushion or by moving into a bad sitting posture to relieve the pain. You sit properly or you lie down. *It's that simple.*

You can actively work on a good sitting posture once any wounds have healed. This is how to sit properly, literally:

- Always sit (yes, always, and don't slouch) in a neutral position and upright (see page 146). To check you are doing this correctly, you can ask someone to take a photo of you from the side. Is your back straight? And look at the line that can be drawn from one ear, down through the shoulder joint to the hip joint: it should be perpendicular to the floor.
- Put two feet on the floor; don't cross your legs or your feet.
- Do not sit tightly against the backrest; you won't be able to sit upright.

## TRAINING TIPS

Sitting isn't as relaxing as it seems. When you sit up straight, you are actually tensing your muscles. Things often go wrong when you give in to that relaxed feeling and start slouching.

Sitting is the new smoking, and sitting for too long is extremely bad for you. Make sure you don't sit for lengthy periods. Set an alarm—set it for every hour as far as I am concerned—and move around, even if you only get up, move your head from left to right and dip through your knees a few times. Try and take at least 250 steps: go pour a glass of water, walk an extra lap around the room with your baby, see whether the mail has arrived, walk to a colleague, or make up any excuse to get out of your seated position. Not only is it good to alternate sitting with moving, but also it prevents your metabolism from slowing down due to being in a resting position for too long. In short, it also helps you lose weight.

Sitting on a gym ball rather than a chair is extremely good for you. Choose a reasonably large gym ball so that you don't have to pull your knees up too high. The gym ball doesn't provide support and will roll away if you don't sit straight the whole time and tense the right muscles. In short, you must stay in control when sitting on a gym ball and you can't cheat. It's also a good idea to move to the left and right a little (movements to keep the pelvis supple) and back and forward. The less time you sit completely still, the better.

Did you know that edema (holding on to fluid) in your feet and legs, for example, can occur and get worse from sitting for a long time? Get off that chair and move around.

## SWITCHBLADE MOTION: BUT NOT IF YOU HAVE A LARGE DIASTASIS

See your body as a switchblade with a top part (your torso and head) and a bottom part (your legs), and imagine the spring motion you can make with it: as if your body is folding in half. It is a good exercise to do when you can stay conscious of your movements, but you shouldn't do this motion without paying attention or coordinating your movements. And you should avoid it completely if you have a large diastasis. When you are lying down and want to get up, first roll onto your side and then get up. That will prevent you from putting any extra pressure on your abdominal muscles.

## Standing

Just like sitting, standing still for too long isn't good for you, either. When you stand still, everything in your body drops to the bottom due to the effect of gravity. Moreover, when you are not doing anything, there is nothing to stimulate your blood circulation. You go into a resting position, which isn't beneficial if it lasts for too long. When you move, you use the muscles around the blood vessels. Because this tightening of the muscle pinches the vessels even more, your blood flow improves. If you stand for over an hour without alternating it with movement, the leg muscles don't pump the blood to the heart properly. This can cause edema or varicose veins. It's also a good idea to stand on your toes a few times, which will activate the muscle pumps in your calves and promote the discharge of fluid from your body.

When you stand straight, your midriff (diaphragm) has a lovely dome shape. It allows you to get the maximum amount of air from the bottom of your lungs. The diaphragm works closely with the pelvic floor. If your diaphragm is constricted because you are leaning forward, for example, your pelvic floor can't function to the full.

This is how to stand properly and look good doing it:

1. Avoid letting your back "hang." When you are tired, you have the tendency to slouch, which creates a hollow lower back and a rounded upper back and pushes your belly forward.
2. Slightly tense your belly using your abdominal muscles. However, you are not supposed to hold in your belly to the extent that it restricts your breath.
3. Make sure your knees aren't "locked."
4. Tense your butt slightly when standing so that your hips tilt forward somewhat.
5. Stand proud: shoulders back slightly and down.
6. When you stand, stand with your legs slightly apart (at hip width) and don't overstretch your knees.
7. Don't "rest" on one hip when standing still. Stay centered and focused.

## THE POSITION OF YOUR FEET AFFECTS YOUR PELVIC FLOOR

Give it a go: stand with your feet pointing inward. Can you feel how your hips tilt and you have less space in your pelvis? It's the same when you stand with your feet pointing outward. So, always pay attention to the position of your feet because, once again, as you can see, everything is connected.

When you stand properly, you use your whole foot. You don't stand on your heel or toes but spread the weight over your entire foot.

# TRAINING TIPS

Imagine you are wearing a pair of pants with a zipper going from your pelvic bone to your belly button that you can zip up tightly from the bottom to the top. This will help you tense the right abdominal, butt, and back muscles. A fun additional fact: your buttocks (which is already an extremely attractive part of the body) will look even better, and it's a healthy way to hold in your belly.

These are bad postures that I often see adopted by women who are recovering from pregnancy:

- **The shoulders move forward.** The breasts are, of course, bigger and heavier when you are breastfeeding. There is, therefore, more weight at the front of your body, and it is a natural, but wrong, response to allow the shoulders to hang forward.

- **An overly rounded upper back.** This is also due to the heavier breasts. You compensate for that weight by rounding your back, but this puts pressure on your vertebrae, so that's not a good idea. The back exercises we do in the BTY training ensure your back gets strong enough to allow you to carry the weight of your breasts with a straight posture. Also make sure you wear a good and comfortable supportive bra.

- **A hollow lower back.** When you carry a load of weight at the front of your body, it is all too tempting to slouch your back, which gives you a hollow lower back. If you do that too often or for too long, the back muscles shorten and there's a significant risk that standing with a hollow lower back will become your new default posture.

- **The muscles running alongside your spine remain constantly tense for too long.** If your back is not strong enough to carry the weight of your breasts and to lift your baby, the muscles running directly along the spine, the paraspinal muscles, will do their absolute best to keep your back straight. Or, in other words, they will continually tighten. That's not a good idea. Muscles can't be tense the entire day. That is why it's important to teach the paraspinal muscles to carry the new weight comfortably without too much strain. For this reason too, it's good to sit on a gym ball. Even by simply breathing and moving your head, for instance, the paraspinal muscles make small movements and become suppler, and it stops them from being tensed in the same position the entire time.

## Lifting

Quickly lifting something without bending your legs, instead bending forward, places you in a strange position with your legs stretched and strains your back. It's something we all do on occasion, but it is not good for you, especially when you are recovering from pregnancy and childbirth. When you lift something incorrectly, you strain your back muscles in the wrong way, you damage your vertebrae, and you are being anything but nice to your pelvis.

This is how to lift properly from a lower level or from the floor:

1. Stand right in front of the object you want to lift.
2. Keep your legs wide and bend through your knees.
3. Lift the object, preferably at chest height, and come up slowly.
4. Pay attention to your powerhouse while lifting; tense your abdominal, back, and pelvic floor muscles; and keep breathing. This gives you stability, but because you keep breathing, you won't put too much pressure on your powerhouse (and, in particular, on the pelvic floor muscles). A plus point: you have done one of your daily squats, which gives you a shapely butt and strong legs.

## TRAINING TIPS

- **Get your child to help you as much as they can.** You could spend the entire day lifting your child, but if, for example, they can stand on their own and hold on to you—making it easier for you to lift them—let them do it. It's good for your body and good for their independence and their body, too.
- **Choose a system of carrying your baby in several positions: on your belly, on your back, and later on your hips.** Regularly alternate the position you carry them in.
- **If you have a prolapse, don't lift your baby too often or carry them for too long on your belly.** When baby is on your belly, you can't take a full XL Breath and you will compensate for that with a different type of breathing, which will put too much pressure on your powerhouse. That pressure will be released at the weakest point, in that case underneath where you have the prolapse.

## Holding Your Baby

Within a year, your baby grows from about 6.6 pounds to 22 pounds, and you are lifting, putting down, and moving around those pounds throughout the day. In short, it's a major workout for your body and it won't surprise you to hear that many health issues after childbirth come from this continual lifting. That is why it's so important to do it the right way and be aware of how you are doing it. These golden lifting rules are good for your neck, back, powerhouse, and . . . thumbs.

## TRAINING TIPS

- **Stand in an active neutral posture (see page 146)** when you want to put baby down or pick them up, and don't ever lean against something (e.g., the side of the bed). It may feel more comfortable, but it causes you to hollow your back and, therefore, puts a massive amount of pressure on your powerhouse. Lift without leaning. Always.

- **Hold your baby as close to your chest as you can.** The closer the weight you are lifting is to your body, the lighter it feels. And close to your chest and belly is by far the nicest place for your baby. When you want to put baby down, hold them with two arms and against your chest. Make sure your head, back, and pelvis form a straight line. Let your head lead you and bend forward, then follow with your back and pelvis. Keep your baby against you for as long as possible; only move them farther away when you have no other choice.

- **Pick up and put down your baby on an exhalation, but do nothing while inhaling.** You should only make strength movements on an exhalation.

- **Alternate sides.** Put down your baby from a different side each time. One time put them down from a left turn, the next from a right turn. Not only should you use this principle when putting your baby down, but also when lifting or picking them up and with all other movements you make with your baby. Don't keep straining the same muscles on the same side.

- **Pay attention to your thumbs.** It sounds crazy, but 1 in 10 women suffer from painful thumbs when they have a baby. It is tempting to tense your hands when you lift your baby because you want to avoid dropping them. But it's not good for you. Pay attention so that you don't strain your thumbs when you lift your baby.

## Toilet position

There are three openings in the middle of your pelvic floor muscles, two of which are used when you go to the bathroom: one for urination (part of the urinary tract) and one to pass stools (the anus). As soon as something passes through your pelvic floor and needs to exit, you tighten or relax those muscles. And now that your pelvic floor deserves some tender loving care, it's a good idea to pay attention to your toilet position so that you don't damage your pelvic floor or impede your recovery. You will also reduce the risk of getting a bladder infection or hemorrhoids.

For a perfect visit to the bathroom:

1. Place both feet flat on the ground, slightly apart, and relax. It's better if you put your feet on a little step (or even better, on a Squatty Potty) so that your knees are slightly raised. The "squatting position" allows your pelvic floor muscles to relax, and you can then urinate and poop until your bowels are completely empty.
2. Are you done? Tense your pelvic floor and relax again.
3. Wipe yourself from the front to back and never the other way around. Now you can get up.

**PATRICK JOHNSON**, posture and coordination expert and Alexander Technique specialist, Amsterdam, The Netherlands

You could see it this way: you don't take on a posture, but your posture is formed by how you tighten your muscles. If you systematically tighten or relax your muscles too much during certain movements or in certain situations, it can cause health issues.

TIPS:

1. **To start with, it is important to figure out which muscles you unconsciously tighten and relax at certain times.** If you are sitting in front of a computer concentrating and you unconsciously move your neck and shoulders toward the screen, for example, that can be bad for your body in the long term.

2. **Be conscious of your body when you rush to your baby.** Do you allow the desire, your emotion, to get to baby as quickly as possible to influence your body posture? Do you run to them with your head pushed forward, your arms outstretched, and with a tense back and shoulders long before you are close to them? If so, ask yourself the question: did it make you faster? And how would you have done it if you had all the time in the world? By thinking about the relationship between emotions and actions, you often realize that you can easily adapt certain things in your lifestyle, which will do wonders for your posture.

3. **If you find it hard to monitor your whole body and how it reacts to certain situations, first focus on your neck and head.** Many things you do to keep your body in a certain position are caused by tightening the neck muscles.

# Breathing

You have been breathing since birth, so what could possibly go wrong? A lot. And that's a shame because your body and your mind benefit greatly from proper breathing. Luckily, it's fairly easy to learn and adopt a new, improved breathing technique. You will notice the difference within just a few weeks!

These are the benefits of a good breathing rhythm for your body and your mind:

**REDUCES STRESS AND, INDIRECTLY, YOUR STRESS HORMONES:** When you are stressed, you often breathe "high up" in your body, without using your belly. That costs your body a lot of energy, even though you won't be aware of it. Your body doesn't have the chance to relax, which causes more tension, resulting in stress in your body and stress in your mind.

**DOESN'T STRAIN YOUR BODY BUT RELIEVES IT:** By breathing incorrectly, you put the wrong kind of pressure on certain body parts. If, for instance, you unconsciously push while breathing, you put pressure on the pelvic floor muscles every time you breathe. When you breathe deeply with your belly, you don't put any extra pressure on your pelvic floor muscles. If you breathe incorrectly, you strain other parts of your body, but a good breathing technique relieves it.

**GIVES YOU MORE ENERGY:** Your body needs oxygen to produce energy. A good breathing technique improves the transportation of oxygen to the mitochondria. These are tiny cell organelles found in almost every cell of our body; you could see them as the cell's energy factory. The more oxygen your body gets, the more efficient the mitochondria are and the more energy they can produce.

**IMPROVES DIGESTION:** When you are stressed, your body is in a type of survival mode. All the energy entering your body is devoted to "surviving." Other processes, such as your digestive system, will get less energy. When you calm down by breathing correctly, you indirectly reactivate your digestive system, which is good for losing weight. Breathing properly to lose weight . . . well, that sounds good to me.

**HAS A DETOXIFYING EFFECT:** You discharge all kinds of unwanted substances from your body through your lymphatic system. The lymphatic system doesn't have its own pump to regulate the supply and discharge of substances; it is activated by moving and breathing. When you move and breathe, you activate your muscles, and they help transport and discharge the lymph fluid when they contract.

**HELPS DEACIDIFY YOUR BODY:** Put simply, you inhale oxygen and exhale $CO_2$. The more $CO_2$ that remains in your body, the greater the negative effect on your body's acidity. In turn, this can influence your hormone levels, and it could make you more susceptible to inflammation, for example.

**PREVENTS AND REDUCES SOME NECK AND HEADACHE ISSUES:** Although shallow breathing seems easier, it's extremely hard work for your body. Your muscles must tense so much that the surrounding muscles often cramp, which can result in neck issues or headaches.

## EVEN YOUR HEART SHIFTS UP WHEN YOU ARE PREGNANT

Your entire respiratory system went through some major changes during your pregnancy. It was harder to breathe, your diaphragm was under stress, and your heart moved over, to give just a few examples. It's no surprise, then, that you have to get used to breathing with an "empty belly" again. Everything in your body must find its place again, and that can take some getting used to. The breathing exercises in the program give you a helping hand with that.

Do the test: Do you breathe in the best possible way? See page 265.

## But . . . How Do You "Breathe Properly" Then?

Basically, there are three types of breathing:

1.  **Chest breathing.** With this type of breathing, the muscles between the ribs contract, meaning your rib cage rises and the space between the ribs increases. The air is sucked into your lungs, as it were. It sounds complicated, but when you see your chest move outward, that is chest breathing. Many, and by this we mean lots and lots of people, breathe by way of chest breathing. This type of breathing is extremely hard work for your body, even if it seems easy to do. It costs a lot more energy than abdominal breathing.

2.  **Abdominal breathing.** With abdominal breathing, you use your belly. Instead of expanding your chest with your rib muscles, you enlarge the chest cavity by lowering your diaphragm. You will see your belly protrude slightly. As women, we may not be keen on seeing that, but it's much better for your body because you only use muscle strength when inhaling and not when exhaling.

3.  **The XL Breathing.** This is the ideal combination of chest and abdominal breathing that is initiated from the belly, which then forms a solid foundation for expanding the lungs. Your lungs can get more air. You mainly use your belly, but your ribs join in and you will feel them move to the side when you take a breath. This

means you use all the available space in your body to take in air. The more space there is for this air, the more the air can spread out and the lower the pressure within your powerhouse. And that's what it's all about: spreading out the pressure to put the least amount of strain on your powerhouse. Moreover, this breathing technique allows your diaphragm to move freely without coming under extreme pressure from above or below.

The air enters the lungs through:

1. **Nasal breathing.** Your nose filters the air, makes it moister (the lungs like that), and warms the air.
2. **Mouth breathing.** It doesn't filter anything, warm anything, or make anything moister, but it is a quick fix to get a large amount of oxygen into your body in one go. If you breathe through your mouth a lot, it could be harder to get rid of a chronic cold and you could snore. Besides that, it gives you a dry mouth, which can cause numerous other issues, such as a sore throat and bad breath.

In short, breathing is vital and breathing correctly helps your body recover. And that is why we start every BTY training session with several focused breathing exercises while you visualize and feel how your pelvic floor rises when you exhale and falls when you inhale.

# XL FUNDAMENTAL: EXERCISE AND TRAINING

We hear it all over the place: sitting is the new smoking, exercise is good for you, and training is part of a healthy lifestyle. Both exercise as well as training impact your body and your mind. They work together and reinforce each other. It is with good reason that exercise and training are the fourth XL Fundamental.

# Exercise

We all move throughout the day but, generally speaking, we don't do enough active exercise or moderately intensive exercise. By moderately intensive exercise, we mean anything that raises your heart rate and quickens your breathing but that still allows you to hold a conversation. Examples include walking up a few stairs, walking at a brisk pace, or cycling fast, but also the daily favorites, such as tidying the house, cleaning, and gardening.

See active exercise as daily maintenance for your body. It's good for your overall fitness, prevents your body from going into "pause mode," and stimulates the blood circulation in your muscles, which gives you a lovely blush and glow on your cheeks.

## BACK TO YOU: THE EXERCISE STANDARD

*Exercise is recovery!*

Exercise every day for at least 30 minutes in a row at moderate intensity.

- This is separate from the training sessions (two to three times a week) and the attention you should give to your posture and to alternating movements after sitting or standing for an hour. Officially, you should move every 20 minutes, but let's be honest, that's simply not feasible when you are at work. That is why we've set it at every hour. That hour is also the maximum.
- If you do this, you will recover to the max, become a better version of yourself, and your posture, daily exercise, and training will reinforce each other. You will really get the synergetic effect of 1 + 1 = 3.

With this program, we use our own minimum standard of exercise. You often read that 150 minutes of exercise a week is enough. It isn't.

## TRAINING TIPS

- Take the stairs.
- Go for a walk (and don't drag your feet) on your lunch break.
- Wear a step counter that alerts you when you need to walk and that tells you how many steps you have done in a day.
- Walk around when you are on the cell phone.
- Take your car less often; only use it if you can't cycle or walk.
- Get into a habit of taking a good daily walk and keep up the pace.

## Walking

Walking is the most well-known form of exercise and something that's nice to do with your baby, too. We aren't talking about walking across the room, but a walk of at least 30 minutes and at a brisk pace.

These are the benefits of a daily 30-minute walk:

**GOOD FOR MUSCLES AND BONES:** Walking actively uses your muscles and strains the bones. Your bones are subjected to a good type of pressure (compression), which makes the bones stronger. You even build up new bone mass.

**GOOD FOR YOUR HEART AND LUNGS.**

**GOOD AGAINST ANXIETY AND DEPRESSION:** There are increasing studies that show that walking has a direct and massive impact on anxiety and depression. In fact, you can reduce anxiety disorders by half if you go for a brisk walk for 30 minutes every day. Walking is therefore good for everyone, but especially for those suffering from postpartum stress, postpartum anxiety, or postpartum depression.

**GOOD FOR YOUR HORMONE AND VITAMIN LEVELS:** Due to the additional daylight you get through your eyes, your body produces extra serotonin, and your skin gets an extra dose of vitamin D.

**AND . . . GOOD FOR YOUR BABY:** It's of course a lot of fun and educational to see the outside world!

## TRAINING TIP: THIS IS HOW YOU KNOW WHETHER YOU ARE EXERCISING OR TRAINING

Can you still easily hold a conversation? If so, you are exercising, not training. I have all too often seen people at the gym who think they are training but, in fact, they are exercising. They do an exercise several times, but they could easily do a few more repetitions, it may be tiring, but that's training. It's those final few exercises that you can just about manage. It is precisely that final bit that pushes you over your limit. Then you are training: you are creating stronger muscles. If it's easy to do, then you are exercising. That's good for you, too, but it doesn't count as one of the two or three intensive training sessions per week.

# Training

Training is hard work. You don't train without effort, and you have to push yourself to your limits. You will enjoy these grueling sessions once you get a taste for them. They will break you and make you. By training you strengthen your muscles, give your body a well-deserved boost of hormones, and it's a massive boost for your ego and your overall appearance.

These are all physical and mental benefits!

1. You develop stronger muscles and more muscle mass.
2. Your bones get stronger.
3. Your metabolism speeds up and you burn more energy, so you lose weight.
4. It can help muscles relax and contract.
5. Your overall fitness levels improve.
6. It lowers your blood pressure.
7. It improves your posture.
8. It improves your mood, even with depression.
9. You produce countless hormones that improve your recovery process.
10. And yes, appearance does matter . . . your figure, skin, and overall appearance will improve!

# 1. You develop stronger muscles and more muscle mass

From a physiological perspective, you tear your muscles when you train. That sounds scary, but it's actually a good thing. Your body instantly starts the recovery process and closes the small muscle tears with new muscle cells. So, in fact, by training you cause a change in the protein production in the muscle tissue and you increase the size of the muscle fiber. So, your muscles grow, and they get stronger. When you start training again after a period of not doing any training (because you were pregnant and needed to recover), you build up new muscle mass fairly quickly. That's a bonus!

# 2. Your bones get stronger

Countless studies have shown that your bones become stronger through training due to the mechanical strain on them. This affects your bone mass and bone structure. The result is an improved resilience of the bones. The so-called remodeling principle can reform or replace the bone. This means that, with intensive training, you ensure your bones adapt to the mechanical strain you put on them during heavy and intensive sport. In other words, because of this remodeling, your bones can get stronger and you prevent osteoporosis (bone decalcification). This will help in the long term. By the time you are a grandma, you will still be living an energetic life!

# 3. Your metabolism speeds up and you burn more energy, so you lose weight

Your body's metabolism converts food and reserve fats into energy. When you do a lot of training, your metabolism speeds up. You burn more fat, even in a resting position. In short, not only do you burn calories when training, but your muscles grow and they burn more fat, even when resting. Two fat burners for the price of one!

And we're not finished yet. Not only do you burn the visible fat in the form of rolls of fat, but you also burn the more harmful fat: the white (yellow) visceral fat. This surrounds the organs and inhibits the organs from doing their job. You also have "good" fat: the brown fatty tissue that helps you burn the bad, white fat. You gain more brown fat through training but also by not spoiling yourself with heat all the time and tolerating a little cold. Therefore, turn down your heat sometimes, take off that warm sweater for an hour on occasion, and finish off with a nice cold shower every so often.

# 4. It can help your muscles relax and contract

It sounds counterintuitive, but sometimes you can get a muscle to completely relax by tensing it for a moment. When you train a muscle, it must contract and then relax again. It seems that sometimes muscles need that tightening so that they can totally relax afterward. Or training shortens the muscles, meaning they can shoot back into the elongated relaxed position all by themselves.

## 5. Your overall fitness levels improve

You increase your lung capacity through training. Lung capacity is the amount of air you inhale and exhale per breath. With an improved lung capacity, you can inhale more air (oxygen) and exhale more "spent" air. You, therefore, inhale more air and can do more with that air. Air is good for your blood circulation, your heart, skin, and all your body parts, in fact. And you will notice it in your overall fitness levels—you won't get out of breath as quickly, you'll be able to handle more, and you get into a positive, upward spiral. You can do more, so you do more, which results in you being able to do even more, and so on.

## 6. It lowers your blood pressure

Your heart's pumping mechanism gets stronger when you train regularly. You need fewer beats to pump the blood around your body. Fewer beats per minute means a lower heart rate. It makes perfect sense, really, because training strengthens your muscles. And your heart is a muscle, after all.

## 7. It improves your posture

We have already spoken extensively about the advantages of good posture, but you need strong muscles to adopt that good posture. You build up the strength in your muscles through training, which means you will be able lift objects easily, carry your baby without harming your body, protect your back from sagging under the influence of gravity, and so on.

## 8. It improves your mood, even with depression

We used to search for salvation in talking and drugs, but increasing studies are now showing that training regularly and adjusting your diet can have a massive effect on your mood.

Training is a must if you have postpartum stress, anxiety, or depression. It won't be easy to get started if you're feeling bad. That makes sense. But if you find the strength to adjust your diet for a month, to rest and do training, you will be giving yourself a massive gift; namely, that your state of mind will be positively affected. Ask someone to do the BTY program with you to get you motivated and give you the push you need. It will really help. But the question is . . . how does it help?

Strength training has a positive effect on your hormones. And some hormones are responsible for stress, anxiety, and depression. Not only that, but also you can let off steam during a workout and empty your head for a while.

## 9. You produce countless hormones that benefit your recovery

Training has a massive effect on your hormone levels. And that is simply because your body is forced to go slightly over its own limit. That places demands on your body, and you need the hormone testosterone for that. Testosterone has a positive effect on muscle development and inhibits the production of the hormone cortisol. Cortisol is a stress hormone; training, therefore, indirectly reduces stress. That, of course, positively affects your mood. So, you can see that hormones are the link between your physical body and your emotions. But, if you work out for too long (i.e., over an hour), you get the opposite effect. In that case, your body starts producing cortisol and it inhibits the production of testosterone.

The production of testosterone during a workout is, therefore, vital for training to succeed because it influences the ratio of testosterone versus cortisol. Studies have shown that this is only achieved through regular training. A single session, or only a couple of sessions and then nothing, won't have that stress-reducing effect. Similarly, if you regularly train in the same way, your body will get used to it and you won't get that testosterone-increasing and cortisol-reducing effect, either. You must, therefore, keep intensifying or varying the training. This BTY program keeps that in mind and ensures you intensify and vary the exercises at the right time.

You produce dopamine when working out. This neurotransmitter is released during sport, and it is a type of happy substance. So, training is even better for you when you need an extra dose of happy feelings (e.g., if you don't feel so comfortable in your mom skin after childbirth). In addition, dopamine gives you a feeling of reward, and you won't feel the need to grab sugary products to give you a pleasurable feeling, for instance. And as if those benefits of dopamine weren't enough, it also increases your memory and your libido.

## 10. Your figure, skin, and overall appearance will massively improve

Enough of the health benefits. Here are the benefits of training that make you feel like a beautiful and fabulous woman again. Training has an antiaging effect and improves blood flow, which gives you a wonderful *blush and glow*. You sweat out all kinds of toxins through your skin. Your body burns fat and you lose weight. Your butt becomes wonderfully rounded and your legs trimmer. The contours in your face will improve, meaning you don't need to use products and brushes to create them. Even though countless creams promise the same, training is really the only miracle worker that exists—your all-in-one solution to *get your sexy back*!

## TRAINING TIPS

Trainer Laurens is, of course, very much in favor of regular training. But there are times when it's not a good idea to really go for it. These times include when:

- **You have injuries that get worse when you train.**
- **You are taking antibiotics.** Antibiotics disrupt the immune system, which can make it harder for your body to recover after intensive exercise. Ideally, you should wait for four days after finishing the course of treatment before starting training again.
- **You have an infection combined with a fever.**
- **You have a burnout.** In that case, your body is already stressed, and adding the stress of training on top will be too much for your body.

But if you can't train, it goes without saying that you can (or "must") still exercise.

# 10 Golden Training Tips

1. **Train with conviction and love.** It's easy to skip your workout when you are a mother because you are busy, busy, busy. And you are, of course, but training is essential to get healthy and stay healthy. And being healthy is good for you and your family. Stop with the excuse of "no time" and make time! You set your own priorities; they are not forced upon you.

2. **Breathe properly and never ever push.** That means that you must pay attention to your breathing every time you exercise. Keep breathing and don't stop. Each time you stop breathing and use that force to push, you put an immense pressure on your pelvic floor, and that's not good.

3. **Train at the right intensity.** You should make the exercises hard enough so that you can just about do them. Not so easy that you're not putting in any effort, but not so hard that you start compensating with other body parts or adopt the wrong posture.

4. **Train your full range of motion: train XL motion.** A muscle is only trained to the max when you train the full range of motion and, therefore, not just a small part of the movement the muscle can make. A well-trained muscle can completely relax (extend) and completely tighten (shorten). When you can do both of these well, you are training with XL impact—your XL motion—and you will see XL results.

    Sometimes your body could have a blockage somewhere or an exercise could hurt from a certain point, meaning you can't manage the full range of motion. In that case, do the exercise as far as you can manage and train the muscles in such a way that you will be able to do the exercise completely in the future.

5. **Listen to your body.** Training costs energy, perseverance, and can be painful at times, but there's a difference between feeling something and feeling pain. Training should never hurt. Genuine pain is your body's way of telling you that you are going too far. The exercise may be too intense for you, or you might be doing it wrong. Figure out what's causing the pain and adjust it.

6. **Start and finish at the same pace.** Maintain the same pace of movement during the entire exercise. There's a reason you chose that pace. Speeding up is often a form of giving up and getting gravity to assist you. So don't do it.

7. **Pay attention to your (correct) posture, not only during training.** This is another reason it's good to use a mirror when working out. You can check whether your posture is still correct. People often "forget" their posture when the going gets tough. That's a waste because you will fail to achieve the purpose of the training.

8. **Remember: quality over quantity.** A training session is only worth doing when you execute the exercises correctly, at the right pace, with the right range of motion, and at the right intensity. If you neglect one of these, then it's at the expense of the quality. And the quality is more important than the frequency. You may not be able to do that 10th repetition; if so, do 9. If that happens often, do the

exercise at a lower level so that you can manage both the quality as well as the quantity.

9. **Don't work out on a full stomach.** If you do, your body will be busy digesting the food, and the training won't go as well or the food will get in the way.

10. **Drink before training.** Make sure you have a good drink about an hour before doing the training. There's little point in drinking during the training session because your body needs time to absorb the fluid to get the benefit. A sip of water can be nice if you have a dry mouth, but a dry mouth probably means that you are breathing through your mouth, and you shouldn't be doing that anyway.

# LET'S GET STARTED: YOUR BTY PROGRAM

ow that you know all about your body, your hormones, your brain, and the impact of the XL Fundamentals, we can really get started with the BTY program. You will recover in 40 weeks, and actually, you'll do a whole lot more than that. In 40 weeks, you will transform yourself into a stronger, heathier, and fitter version of yourself—and without any leftover damage from the pregnancy and childbirth!

## The Back To You Program Consists of Three Phases

**1. BACK (0–6 WEEKS):** You take a little step back. Right now, it's about getting rest and making a connection: a connection with your baby and a connection with your new role as mother. The exercises focus on the connection between your mind and your powerhouse.

**2. TO (7–24 WEEKS):** You gradually pick up your "normal" life again. You go back to work, to your social life, to yourself. The physical exercises work toward your stability and mobility. With the nonworkout, we work on your inner you and help you get back to the "normal" world in the process.

**3. YOU (25–40 WEEKS):** You are increasingly becoming your "new you" and finding your own strength. The exercises work intensively on that new you so that you will be healthier, stronger (both mentally as well as physically), and in better shape. You will become your new YOU! Or perhaps even a better version of yourself than ever before.

## And Each Phase Consists of:
- Practical matters: the information you want to know in this phase
- Tips and tricks from the experts for your body and your emotions
- Your Personal Training Program: the BTY blocks:
  - Complete workouts (including suggestions for adjustments to take into account different conditions that you may be experiencing)
  - Exercises, challenges, and tips for the XL Fundamentals
  - Your diary (track your progress! Wow!)
  - Each block lasts three weeks. The first training session in a block is a self-test, which you use to you learn how to adjust the program to your body to get the most out of it. Because with recovery, there is no one-size-fits-all.

## With Each BTY Workout, You Can Expect:

- You will get an explanation of what we do, when we do it, and why we do it.
- Which exercises you'll be doing this week in words and images, portrayed by the BTY stick woman. If you'd rather see a live-action demonstration, then open your BTY app and watch the video that will help you through the whole training session.
- Your workout is mom-proof. It's fast and efficient and filled with special BTY features:
    - XL motion training and a focus on the right pressure distribution in your pelvic floor muscles and the rest of your powerhouse.
    - XL breathe yourself ready for your training. Get rid of those restrictive muscle knots and overly tight muscles.
    - BTY Kegel exercises and/or releasing trigger points: bye-bye, problems and hello, fun!
    - Many of the cooling-down exercises also give you a good dose of mindfulness.

## The XL Fundamentals

- Provide challenges and things that are fun to try and can have a massive impact on your health, looks, and recovery.
- You don't have to follow all these tips and do all the exercises. Read them and pick a few that you like the idea of and that suit you. One thing's for sure: they are often very small adjustments to your lifestyle, yet they will give you major XL benefits.
- Try to do your chosen XL Fundamentals for the three weeks during the entire block.

# The First Training Session of a New Block

During your three-week BTY block, you do the same exercises for three weeks. This method enables you to teach your muscles to adopt the specific postures and makes the muscle groups nice and firm, strong, and stable. Because you do the same exercises for three weeks, you won't even have to think about them at a certain point; you can do them at any time, which is convenient. Those three weeks are just short enough so that your body doesn't get too used to the exercises and become "lazy."

Before you can run on almost automatic pilot, you have an extra step to do in the first training session of the block. You have to test yourself. This takes time and energy, but these self-tests make all the difference. They help you find the right level, and identify the blockages in your body and get rid of them, which will help you tremendously!

**TAKE NOTE:** You don't have to do a self-test during the "Back" phase. These exercises are very gentle and suitable for everyone.

## During the self-test (first training session of the new block), you determine:

- Your starting level
- Whether you need to activate and/or loosen any muscles, and if so, which ones
- The points of your posture you need to pay attention to

# SELF-TEST: FIRST TRAINING SESSION OF THE BLOCK

**STEP 1:** Open your BTY app and do this block's workout for the first time.

**STEP 2:** Film yourself during the training; by watching yourself you can analyze your mistakes. Film yourself from the front and then the side by turning after a few repetitions.

**STEP 3:** Do the first exercise at level 1, or the level you reached before if you've done this exercise already. Watch your video and answer these questions:

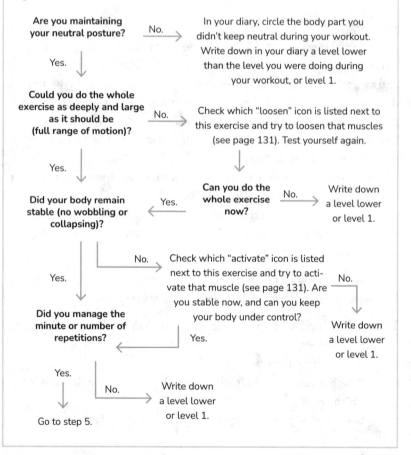

Are you maintaining your neutral posture? — No. → In your diary, circle the body part you didn't keep neutral during your workout. Write down in your diary a level lower than the level you were doing during your workout, or level 1.

Yes. ↓

Could you do the whole exercise as deeply and large as it should be (full range of motion)? — No. → Check which "loosen" icon is listed next to this exercise and try to loosen that muscles (see page 131). Test yourself again. ↓

Can you do the whole exercise now? — No. → Write down a level lower or level 1.

Yes. ←

Yes. ↓

Did your body remain stable (no wobbling or collapsing)?

Yes. ↓ No. → Check which "activate" icon is listed next to this exercise and try to activate that muscle (see page 131). Are you stable now, and can you keep your body under control? — No. → Write down a level lower or level 1.

Yes. ↓

Did you manage the minute or number of repetitions? ← Yes.

Yes. ↓ No. → Write down a level lower or level 1.

Go to step 5.

**STEP 4:** Can you proudly say yes to all five questions? If so, do the test at a higher level and ask yourself the same questions again.

**STEP 5:** Write down level 3 next to all exercises that you could do well at level 2 on all points.

**STEP 6:** You have been introduced to this block's workout by doing this self-test. Check you have properly filled in everything in your workout schedule so that you can join in during the coming weeks.

**STEP 7:** Put the results of your self-test in your workout. Fill in:

- **Your starting level for each exercise.**

- **Whether you first need to activate and/or loosen muscles.**

- **During which exercise you need to pay extra attention to a certain aspect of your (neutral) posture.** Put a circle around that part of the stick woman.

- **Whether you need to pay attention to your pace of movement with a certain exercise.**

- **Whether each day, alongside your training, you need to activate, roll, stretch, or demand functionality.** (This will be the result of the self-test you will do for the exercises you haven't been able to do so far, enabling you to see whether activating or loosening helps.)

- **Also, fill in your starting data for that block on page 291 before starting a new phase.** It will give you insight into your progress.

## IN YOUR CALENDAR AND ON YOUR LIST OF PRIORITIES

### EVERY DAY

- BTY Kegel exercises (see page 139). Do them at any point during the day; they take less than a minute ;-). They can help prevent and reduce all symptoms in your lower body and will give you more sexual pleasure. Try to do them three times a day.
- If during the self-test you find that you need to activate, relax, or loosen certain muscles, then do that first before doing the exercise next time and on the days you are not training. That will prevent stiffness and keep your muscles active and/or allow them to relax. When doing the self-test for a specific muscle group, read what you can do to ensure you can properly tighten and relax this muscle. Do it for a few days and you will experience a world of difference, and not only when you are training!

### THREE TIMES A WEEK

- Your workouts. Add them to your calendar, schedule them in, and make them a priority. You and your body deserve it.

### WHAT SUITS YOU AND WHEN

- Read the XL Fundamental tips and challenges. See what things you like the look of and give them a go. They are "little things" that can have a massive impact. Try them for three weeks. Those three weeks are long enough for you to figure out whether they work for you, whether you like doing them, and whether you notice any results.

# Just Gave Birth or Gave Birth Years Ago

The BTY program is suitable for everyone. If you have just given birth, you can do all the exercises in the "Back" phase, even if you still have a large diastasis, prolapse, or had a cesarean section. They are safe, but always listen to your body. You may be able to feel them, but they shouldn't be painful.

If you have given birth longer than six weeks ago, you can skip Block 1 and do Block 2 in one week instead of three. Therefore, after one week you move onto the "To" phase. If you have just given birth, you can start the second phase once your physician or midwife has given you your final checkup and the go-ahead to pick up your normal life again. That will be around six weeks after the birth.

# The Training Sessions after Your Self-Test

Only the first session of a new block is a self-test. After that, you can get on with it . . .

- Open your BTY app and join in with this block's workout for the first time.
- If, when you did the self-test, you discovered that rolling your muscles loose or activating them helped, then pause the video at a certain point. Roll your muscles loose and then start the video again.
- Do the exercise at your starting level, but if you think you can do a higher level after a few training sessions, go for it!
- Always pay attention to your posture and breathing, and we mean always.
- Don't do the exercises too quickly. You don't want to get the power from gravity or from sweeping your body upward but from pure, concentrated muscle strength.
- It's okay if you can feel the exercises, but they shouldn't hurt. If you feel pain, stop doing the exercise. It's a different matter if the pain is something you already had. Then you can continue the exercise because it's not the cause of the pain. But get any symptoms checked by a physician or physiotherapist. You shouldn't be in pain, after all, and it shouldn't get worse during the training.

# Your Results (After a Couple of Weeks)

After a couple of weeks, you will already notice some significant results. Your abdominal muscles will be nicely back together, your pelvic floor will be stronger, and you will feel fitter and more powerful overall. Keep track of your progress in your diary. Read it regularly and the results will amaze you. Enjoy the well-deserved pride in yourself!

# When Are You Recovered?

You are never really finished with training and following a healthy lifestyle. Training with the XL Fundamentals will have an enormous impact on your body, your looks, your mind, and your hormones. In fact, following this healthy lifestyle could even result in you having to take less medication, an increase in your mental stability, and so on.

There is a point, however, when you will be "back to normal"—a time when your hormones are balanced again, your muscles have recovered, and you feel like a strong woman again. When exactly that is depends on various factors: whether you eat healthily, sleep enough, and relax during the day; whether your posture is good; the levels of stress you've experienced; how well you manage the pelvic floor muscle exercises; whether you've been able to follow the training sessions; and many more factors. One person simply recovers more quickly than another, and it can also differ with each pregnancy. One woman may be completely recovered after nine months; another may take one or two years. Accept this fact and simply do what you can. After all, you can't do any more than that.

You can follow the BTY program for as long as it takes for you to get completely Back To You!

# ACTIVATING, LOOSENING, AND DEMANDING FUNCTIONALITY OF THE MUSCLES

Make sure you concentrate because what you are about to read can have a major impact on your body—from "pains that are part of life," such as lower back pain that restricts you from doing certain movements, to a stiff neck that makes a cracking noise or legs that can't bend beyond a certain point, etc. These issues are often easily solved by giving your muscles the *tender loving care* they need by activating, loosening (followed by stretching), and "demanding functionality."

First a technical term: *demanding functionality* is using a muscle to let it know what it should be doing.

These muscle treatment methods are the way to:
- Reduce or get rid of pain
- Enable you to make all movements without being restricted
- Deliver improved muscle performance
- Recover better and quicker

# If Your Muscle Function Is Restricted

You use your muscles to make movements. If your muscles are restricted (because they are too short or due to stiff structures such as the capsules and ligaments around the joint), you will not be able to make the full movement. Or, in other words, your XL motion will be restricted. You won't be able to do a movement properly, or you will unconsciously adjust the movement (compensate). That compensation could cause other issues. And there is another disadvantage to restricted muscle function. If a muscle is too tight (shortened), the opposite muscle will lengthen. In short, neither muscle will be doing what it is supposed to be doing. On top of that, restricted muscle function can have a detrimental effect on your training results. If you find that you can't do the movements completely or comfortably during the training, go to a physiotherapist.

Your muscles work at their best when:
- They are not restricted in their XL motion, from completely relaxed to completely tightened.
- They are not stiff because they have been tensed the entire day.
- They are not so weak that they can't perform their function.
- The muscle-brain connection is at its best.

# Activating and Loosening Do Wonders for Your Muscles

There are simple methods you can use to give your muscles exactly what they need.

**STEP 1:** Find out which muscle has restricted function.

**STEP 2:** Check whether:
- The muscle is "activated." If not, you need to activate the muscle.
- Is it restricted by knots/cramps (stiffness)? If so, you need to loosen the knots by rolling them loose (followed by stretching regularly and/or demanding functionality).

**STEP 3:** Make sure your muscles continue to benefit from being activated, loosened, or stretched.

## Step 1: This Is How You Find Out Which Muscle's Function is Restricted

You start each training block with a self-test. You do the new exercises from the new block for the first time, but you will try out various things to determine your level and the extent of your recovery. Because we know which muscles you will be using during the exercises, we also know which potential restrictions the muscle could have. That is why we also get you to see whether the exercise works better if you activate, roll, or stretch the muscle first. The icons listed by the exercises will show you the way.

## Step 2: Activate and/or Loosen?

**IF YOUR MUSCLES (NO LONGER) DO WHAT YOU WANT TO THEM TO DO: ACTIVATE THEM.** If you cannot do the movement properly, see whether it helps to activate your muscles. It could seem like your muscles aren't "switched on" or they refuse to do what you want at a certain point. It's as if they are not listening to you. You slump or your knees collapse inward, you waver, you can't go deep enough, you notice you can't go deeper after a few repetitions, or you lose control in some other way. In short, your movement is too small or gets increasingly smaller. If that's the case, activating your muscles will help. If you still don't have control of your muscles after activating them, they are too weak and they need more training. Read how you activate your muscles on page 131.

**IF YOU FEEL PAIN AT A SPECIFIC POINT OR STIFFNESS IS RESTRICT-ING YOU FROM MAKING A MOVEMENT: ROLL THEM LOOSE.** If you feel something pulling or feel a painful spot while doing the movement, try loosening the muscle by rolling it. You may have muscle knots that are restricting you.

The knots might not be painful, but you notice you can't move past a certain point and the muscle doesn't seem to stretch any farther. Or that point is stiff. You can try to roll the muscle loose.

A muscle could also be overactive. If you continually use that muscle and it cramps and shortens, you will feel that as stiffness. You can help those stiff muscles by rolling them loose. Stiff muscles not only inhibit your freedom of movement but also can cause injuries. Read how you roll your muscles loose on page 131.

## Step 3: Make Sure the Effect Lasts

You will notice an instant effect after activating or loosening a muscle! Pains will be reduced or even gone, you can make the movement you couldn't do before, or you feel suppler.

Wonderful. But, of course, you want that effect to last. See the activation or loosening as a "quick fix." Consider stretching, or demanding functionality and the activation after loosening, as necessary "aftercare." And this is how you do it . . .

**ACTIVATE: ALWAYS AFTER ROLLING A MUSCLE LOOSE.** A muscle could be less stable after loosening it. After rolling, activate it straight away to kick-start your stability. Mobility without stability is asking for trouble in the form of injuries. See it this way: by rolling the muscle loose, the muscle will have relaxed to such a degree that it needs to be "woken up" by activating it.

**DEMANDING FUNCTIONALITY: RIGHT AFTER ACTIVATION AND DURING THE DAY.** After activating or loosening the muscles, you should remind your muscles what they should be doing during the day so that they don't "forget." Do the movement that you couldn't manage or was restricted (before you activated or loosened it) and hold the position. If you still can't manage it, try activating or loosening it again. After a while, you won't have to do it any more or less frequently.

Your muscle has a type of "memory." This means that, at a certain point, the muscle will be able to do what it's supposed to and won't become restricted again. An example: imagine you couldn't do the squat deep enough because your butt muscle was too short. You rolled the butt muscle loose and then you could manage it. After that, it's important to go into a deep squat regularly and throughout the day. You squat to remind your butt muscle of the stretch it should be able to make at the deepest point.

**STRETCH: REGULARLY THROUGHOUT THE DAY.** If your muscle is looser after rolling it, you want it to stay that way. A loosened muscle is a muscle that has released any cramping and is relaxed, which means it can elongate again. To ensure your muscle doesn't forget that it should be long and relaxed, you should stretch it regularly and throughout the day to remind it.

# Activating Your Muscles: This Is How You Do It

After "waking up" or "switching on" your muscle by activating it, you get a better grasp on using that muscle. It is as if the connection between your brain and the muscle becomes more active. That seems complicated, but it's little more than identifying the inactive muscle and drumming, tapping, rubbing, making circles, or hitting it several times in a row for 15 to 20 seconds. You wake up your muscle with your hand!

# Loosening Your Muscles: This Is How You Do It

You need a foam roller or a hard ball to roll your muscles loose.

You use the foam roller to loosen larger areas. Place the foam roller on the floor or against the wall in a position that allows you to roll it over or against the muscle while applying light pressure. Try rolling ¾ inch forward and ½ inch back. Did you find a painful spot? If so, hold the roller there while applying light pressure. Don't forget to breathe properly throughout so that you don't put any unnecessary pressure on your powerhouse. After rolling, you will instantly feel your muscle relax.

You use the hard ball when you want to put extra pressure on a specific, smaller area or a deeper spot you can't reach with a large foam roller, such as your neck. When you want to loosen one specific spot (the knot), place the ball so that you can roll it precisely over the knot. Instead of lying on the ball, you could clamp the ball between your body and the wall. Then apply light pressure by moving up and down. When you want to treat your neck, your head will be in the way, preventing you from clamping the ball between your neck

# ACTIVATING MUSCLES

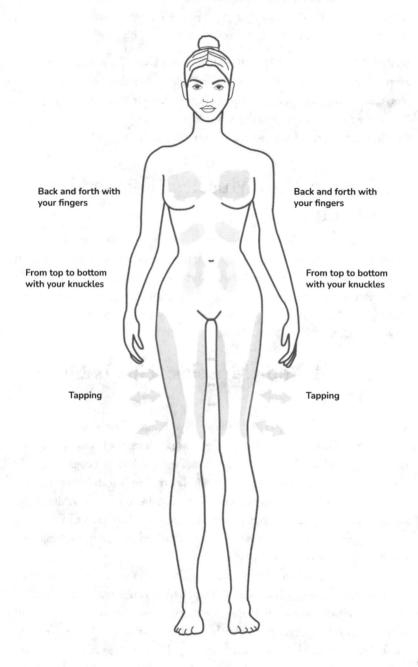

Back and forth with
your fingers

Back and forth with
your fingers

From top to bottom
with your knuckles

From top to bottom
with your knuckles

Tapping

Tapping

Finish activating by demanding functionality of the muscle—putting the muscle to good use!

and the wall. You can solve that by first placing a (foam) block against the wall before clamping the ball between the block and the painful spot in your neck.

Rolling muscles loose also activates your lymph circulation, which releases waste products. Make sure you drink enough water so your body can get rid of those waste products.

**TAKE NOTE:** It is not good to roll your muscles too often or too hard. You could become sore or damage the muscle. To prevent you from needing to roll too often, it's important that you always stretch and/or demand functionality after rolling, and that you do it regularly during the following days.

## GOLDEN TIP! MUSCLE KNOTS . . .

You could have troublesome knots that restrict you and are painful. Did you know that it is often highly effective to find that knot with your thumb and then put pressure on it for a few seconds? After a while, you will suddenly feel the knot soften and disappear. If you feel the pressure radiating from the spot when you put pressure on it, then you are not on a muscle but a nerve.

Many people suffer from lower back pain or stiffness. This method can often offer a lot of relief or even get rid of any issues! Ask someone to loosen the knots around your lower vertebrae and your entire hip region, including your buttocks. Get them to put a lot of pressure on the knots so that they relax. Stiff butt muscles can also cause lower back issues!

This method shows us the latest insights: sometimes you need to put pressure on a muscle to enable it to relax.

# Stretching: This Is How You Do It

After loosening your muscles, you must finish off by stretching to keep the muscles elongated and relaxed. You can stretch anytime and anywhere, and you can prevent issues by regularly stretching tight muscles. The principle of stretching is amazingly simple: put your body in a position so that you feel the muscle start to pull. Slowly move your body up and down around the point until you feel the stretch. Always stretch for 20 seconds; that's how long a muscle needs to relax.

There is, in fact, another benefit to the leg stretches we do in the BTY program: the muscles on the inside of your legs are connected to the pelvic floor. If you don't stretch these well, you can't properly activate your pelvic floor. Not only that, but also tight inner leg muscles that pull on the pelvic floor will prevent you from being able to train the pelvic floor muscles properly. You won't be able train your pelvic floor muscles separately from your leg muscles.

## DIASTASIS OR CESAREAN SECTION? DON'T STRETCH THE VERTICAL ABDOMINAL MUSCLES!

If you have a large diastasis or had a cesarean section and are not fully recovered, be careful with stretching the vertical abdominal muscles too far (e.g., bending over backward)! Only stretch upward in a straight line and avoid leaning backward.

# Demanding Functionality: This Is How You Do It

After activating or rolling (and possibly followed by stretching), you want the muscle to know what it should do in its elongated, stretched form so that it doesn't forget that movement. This is called *demanding functionality*. You stand, lie, or sit in the position you had trouble with during the self-test. Find the farthest point and hold it there. Don't move up and down as with stretching, but hold one position. Teach that muscle what it's supposed to be doing! Do this regularly during the day and the coming days for as long as you need to until your muscle has gotten used to it.

## TRAINING TIP

Once you have grasped the trick of activating, loosening (followed by stretching), and demanding functionality, you may ask yourself why no one has told you this before. Everyone is different, explains Laurens. He describes one woman who, after only three minutes of following these guidelines, could tilt her pelvis freely and slept for the first time without lower back pain. Another client always had neck pain, which she couldn't get rid of even after seeing numerous physiotherapists. She can now activate and loosen her muscles and her neck pain is gone.

You need to come to grips with the process and become adept at it, but it will be great help once you do. Once you grasp these techniques, you can also help others get rid of their muscle knots. You will gradually develop a feel for it, and you will get better at understanding what your body needs when you feel something.

Of course, the aim is to get to a point that your muscles no longer need the tender loving care of activation or loosening but can function without any preparation. You do that by training. That's how you make your muscles more stable and improve the blood flow in the muscles.

# YOUR DAILY PELVIC FLOOR EXERCISES

In your BTY program, we train your entire powerhouse and we gradually increase the pressure (also the pressure distribution in your powerhouse). It will gradually get more difficult and you will gain more control of your powerhouse and, therefore, of your pelvic floor muscles. And those latter muscles need more training besides those three times a week. And that's what your daily BTY Kegel exercises are for.

# How the Training Program Builds Your Pelvic Floor Muscles

We build things up gradually in your BTY training sessions. During Back, the emphasis is on making the brain connection with your pelvic floor. During To, we focus on strengthening the muscles. And in You, you learn to make your pelvic floor muscles work for you in all situations, even while jumping. Because we build this up gradually and the program lasts for long enough for you to regain the strength in your pelvic floor (your pelvic floor muscles need more than a few weeks to recover), you can prevent incontinence (also at a later age), prevent symptoms such as pain or a feeling of pressure on your pelvic floor, and increase your sexual pleasure. So, there are plenty of reasons to train this muscle group several times a day.

And the best bit is, you can do this anywhere and anytime, and it doesn't cost you any time.

## YOUR PELVIC FLOOR MUSCLES: WHERE ARE THEY? WHAT DO THEY FEEL AND LOOK LIKE?

To train a muscle, you first have to know what it feels like when you tense and relax it. And that's not the easiest thing to do with these muscles. That is why step 1 of the training is to find your pelvic floor muscles. Pick one of the following tips that you like the look of or try them all.

1. **Feel your pelvic floor muscles while urinating.** Try to stop the urine halfway through urinating. Concentrate on the muscles you use for that. They are your pelvic floor muscles. Don't do this often because it's not good for you to stop and then carry on urinating. It's fine to do it once to locate your muscles, but don't make a habit of it. When you urinate, you should completely empty your bladder!

**NOTE:** For the next exercises, empty your bladder before trying them out. You could develop a disrupted urination reflex if you have a full bladder. Not only that, but an empty bladder will help you relax and make it easier for you to feel your pelvic floor muscles.

2. **Embrace your finger with your pelvic floor muscles.** Insert a clean finger into your vagina and try to "embrace" your finger. You use your pelvic floor muscles to do that.

3. **Practice with your partner or a dildo.** If you are already having penetrative sex, then you could try to "clamp" the penis or dildo. Not only will you locate your pelvic floor muscles, but you and your partner will enjoy it, too. Make sure you tense and relax—don't keep clamping.

4. **Feel how a dildo goes in and out while breathing.** You could also insert a dildo about 2 inches into your vagina and consciously breathe in and out. If you have a good connection between your pelvic floor muscles and your breathing, you will feel how the muscles respond to your breathing. The dildo will be pushed out on an inhalation and pulled into your vagina by your pelvic floor muscles when you exhale. By doing this a few times, you will become more aware of the connection between your breathing and your pelvic floor muscles.

5. **View your pelvic floor muscles.** This can help you understand which muscles we are talking about, especially for women who are visually oriented. Lie down with a few pillows under your back and head so that you can see between your legs using a hand mirror. Try to tense your pelvic floor muscles. As soon as you see your vagina closing, your anus tensing, and your perineum (the region between your vagina and anus) pulling upward slightly, you know you have found your pelvic floor muscles.

6. **Not ready to touch or see yourself yet? Blow up a balloon.** This test is only so that you can feel where your pelvic floor muscles are and how they are connected to your breathing. Don't repeat this daily because it would put too much pressure on your muscles. Sit down with your feet on the floor and concentrate on your perineum. Blow up the balloon a little, just until you see the shape of a balloon appearing—so, until you feel resistance. If you are doing it right, you will feel your pelvic floor muscles pushing

your perineum downward when you inhale, and they will rise again when you take the balloon out of your mouth and exhale. Now try to do the same thing without the balloon.

If you still have trouble finding your pelvic floor muscles after following these tips, then go to a pelvic floor therapist so that they can help you. Pelvic floor exercises are incredibly good for you, but they can have the opposite effect if you don't do them correctly.

# Daily BTY Kegel Exercises

The BTY Kegel exercise is a basic exercise that you should do three times a day for the rest of your life. It is a variation of the Kegel exercise, named after gynecologist Dr. Arnold Kegel, whereby you tense and relax your pelvic floor muscles. In the BTY program, we combine this exercise with active breathing and a gentle massage to activate your lymph circulation. That gentle massage gives the pump in your pelvic floor's lymphatic system an extra stimulus.

## BTY Kegel Exercise in the "Back" Phase

To do the Kegel exercises correctly, you first need to have a good connection with your pelvic floor. That will prevent you from tightening other surrounding muscles, and it makes sure that you only train your pelvic floor muscles. It is vital that you do this consciously. That is what will make all the difference!

In these weeks, the BTY Kegel exercises take a little extra time, but in the "To" and "You" phases you don't need to do the connection exercises. You can simply get on with the BTY Kegel exercises wherever you are.

### Step 1: Warm up for your BTY Kegel exercises

1. Find a nice place to sit, lie, or stand and make sure you have a neutral posture.
2. Close your eyes and visualize your powerhouse as a balloon.
3. Feel how the balloon gets bigger as you take a gentle XL Breath (see pages 106–107) and smaller when you exhale.
4. Be aware of the changes in pressure and how the pressure is distributed in the balloon. Can you feel how the pressure is distributed in your belly, back, pelvic floor muscles, and diaphragm? Can you feel the "balloon" between your ribs and your belly slowly getting bigger and then smaller?

### Step 2: The BTY Kegel exercise

1. Make sure your bladder is empty; lie flat on the floor, sit, or stand in a neutral posture. Inhale deeply.
2. On an exhalation, tense your pelvic floor muscles for 3 seconds while using your hands to gently rub/massage from your side to your middle. This stimulates your lymph circulation even more.
3. Then, relax your pelvic floor muscles for at least 3 seconds. It's vital that you relax for the same length of time you tensed the muscles. This is unlike when you train other muscles, such as your abdominal muscles, and you want to keep feeling the tension. Relaxation is much more important for your pelvic floor muscles. If you don't do that, you may develop health issues.
4. Do steps 1 through 3 ten times but alternate the massaging action around your belly with a massaging action from your knees toward your groin.

**TAKE NOTE:** If you've had a cesarean section, massage only your legs until the physician says it's okay for you to massage your belly as well.

### Step 3: The bonus BT Kegel exercise

End your exercise by inhaling deeply and then exhaling. At the final part of the exhalation (when your belly becomes flatter), tense your pelvic floor muscles tightly for 1 second, very tightly and very briefly.

In the second block of "Back" (Weeks 4–6), you will first try to increase the 1-second pump actions you did in the first three weeks up to 3 seconds, without losing the tension in your pelvic floor muscles. But, if it is painful, go back to 1 second or perhaps try 2 seconds. Training your pelvic floor muscles shouldn't be painful.

> It's a great idea to start these BTY Kegel exercises right after childbirth, with the short, pumping actions. That will prevent the brain-pelvic floor connection from weakening. If you have had a tear or incision, it's perfectly normal for you to feel the stitches or the skin around the vagina pulling when you tense your pelvic floor muscles.

## BTY Kegel Exercise (in "To," "You," and for the Rest of Your Life)

This exercise should become your best friend for life. In the BTY program, we gradually increase the number of seconds you do the BTY Kegel exercise from 3 to 5. Because you should tighten the muscles only on an exhalation (if you tighten them while inhaling, you put even more pressure on your pelvic floor, and that is precisely what you don't want), you never do the BTY Kegel exercise for longer than 5 seconds. It's very hard and almost unnatural to exhale for longer than that anyway. The more you do the exercise, the easier it will become and the easier it will be to do it every day without losing any time. In fact, when you make a habit of it, you will almost naturally start doing it more times a day. And even more important, when you are in a situation when you need to tighten your pelvic floor muscles, they will do it all by themselves. Think of when you sneeze, lift something heavy, or during sex.

Don't get worried about all the steps that follow. Once you grasp how to do the exercise, you'll see it's extremely easy to follow and it will give you major benefits.

1. Take a deep XL Breath (see pages 106–107), then take a moment to think about the fact you are going to do the BTY Kegel exercise.
2. During an exhalation, tense your pelvic floor muscles really hard. You decide how long you do it for.
3. Inhale with completely relaxed pelvic floor muscles. When you exhale, tense them again for the number of seconds you are exercising at now.
4. Do this 3 times a day, 10 repetitions each. That's it. By repeating this exercise several times a day, you will have amazing results within a month to a month and a half!

## TRAINING TIP

You could see your pelvic floor as a big pump for your lymphatic system. The BTY Kegel exercises activate your pelvic floor, which stimulates this pump and, therefore, automatically stimulates your lymph drainage. But if, at the same time, you rub your hands over your belly toward your pelvic floor or between your legs toward your pelvic floor, then you activate it even more. Get into a habit of doing this when you are somewhere suitable. Rubbing between your legs while standing in the line at the checkout is not such a good idea, after all ;-)

## Golden Rules for the BTY Kegel Exercises

The BTY Kegel exercises will give you so many benefits in the short and long term, but you have to do them correctly; otherwise you could harm your body. Therefore:

1. Tense your muscles only during an exhalation.
2. Make sure you tighten your muscles for the same amount of time as you relax them! This is extremely important.
3. Only tighten your pelvic floor muscles—not your butt, leg, or abdominal muscles.
4. Every three weeks, check whether you have muscle knots in your vagina (see page 143). If so, you must remove the knots first before actively tensing the muscles. You don't want to make the knots (active muscles) worse by tensing them even more.
5. If it hurts, then you are tightening the muscles for too long and you should reduce the amount of time you are doing it for.

## Variations for Full Control

During the program, you will encounter two variations: you will be doing the BTY Kegel exercises while walking and jumping. These variations will give you increasingly more and better control over your pelvic floor muscles in all situations. You will find these variations in the XL Fundamentals during weeks 25–27 and 31–33 of your program.

## THIS IS HOW YOU KNOW YOU ARE TENSING ONLY YOUR PELVIC FLOOR MUSCLES (OR WHETHER YOU ARE SECRETLY USING OTHER MUSCLES)

Lie flat on the floor, without a pillow under your head, and place your hands on your belly. Tense your pelvic floor muscles. Use your hand to feel whether you are tensing your abdominal muscles. Make sure you don't tense your back or leg muscles at the same time. One way to check whether you are also tightening your butt muscles is by tensing your pelvic floor muscles while sitting down. If you are tensing your butt, you will rise up slightly. Try it and you'll feel the difference. You shouldn't rise up. You really need to relax your butt muscles.

## PAIN WHILE DOING THE BTY PELVIC FLOOR EXERCISES

These exercises shouldn't hurt. If they do, it means your pelvic floor muscles are either over- or underactive. If you feel you are unable to "activate" your muscles, you are doing the exercises but don't really feel anything, or your legs are moving or trembling, then you probably have underactive muscles and you are not tensing the pelvic floor muscles. Go back to the beginning and find your pelvic floor muscles (see page 26).

If you have overactive pelvic floor muscles, you will find knots in that area. Those knots are the result of too much tension and too much stress on the muscles. The pain is the result of these knots combined with tensing too much. You can read how to get rid of knots in your pelvic floor below.

## DISCOVER TRIGGER POINTS ON THE PELVIC FLOOR

### LINDSEY VESTAL, MS, occupational therapist and pelvic floor expert, New York, USA

You can have *trigger points* (knots) in all muscles; therefore, also in your pelvic floor muscles. It is vital to find out whether you have knots in your pelvic floor muscles. Those knots can cause issues when urinating, with your bowel movements, and with your sexual pleasure. In addition, when doing certain exercises, such as the Kegel exercises, your internal trigger points could harm your body. Too few people know about this or do anything about it.

You can go to a pelvic floor specialist and get examined for trigger points, but you can also find out whether you have these overactive muscle knots by doing this test. You do this test inside your vagina. The vagina contains 16 muscles, and if you only examine the outside, you will only feel two of them. Depending on the result, other exercises from the BTY program will be important for you.

### THE TEST

1. Wash your hands (don't forget to clean under your nails) and use a natural lubricant.
2. Insert your index finger into your vagina up to the second knuckle.
3. Tense your pelvic floor muscles and try to "embrace" your finger.

## THE ANALYSIS: ARE YOU DOING THE TEST CORRECTLY?

1. You should feel your finger pull upward slightly, toward your head. If you don't feel it, try it a few more times until you do.
2. Analyze what you feel: can you feel four sides around your finger? Or only two—for example, the front and back or only the sides? If you can't feel all four sides, do it a few more times until you can feel all four sides coming against your finger and feel all four sides "lifting" your finger.

## THE ANALYSIS: WHAT DO YOU FEEL?

Did you feel any pain or a pulling sensation on one of the sides? If so, you probably have overactive muscles and, therefore, trigger points.

## TRIGGER POINTS? RELEASE THEM FIRST BEFORE DOING THE KEGEL EXERCISES

If you have trigger points, then you should wait before doing any Kegel exercises that involve you tensing your pelvic floor muscles. You are only allowed to do the Kegel exercises when you can train them in the full range of motion. The muscles are already too tenses and the last thing you want to do is train those muscles so that they tense even more (become overactive).

## THIS IS HOW TO RELEASE YOUR TRIGGER POINTS

Before doing the Kegel exercises, you need to release your trigger points. You can get a pelvic floor specialist to show you how, or you can do it yourself. Buy a therapeutic vibrator. They are thin, long, and S-shaped, and when you insert the vibrator into your vagina, it looks like you have a handle sticking out which you can use to "steer." And that is exactly what you do: because you know the whereabouts of the trigger point, you can use the point of the vibrator to locate it. Massage the area around it and keep the point on the knot so that it can relax. If you can't find the S-shaped version, you can also use a different vibrator, as long as it has a small curve at the end and is thin so that you can get to the trigger point as accurately as possible without touching the whole vagina.

Massage the trigger points frequently and do the test regularly to see whether your overactive muscle knots, the trigger points, are gone. You can start doing the Kegel exercises once they are gone.

# THE CORRECT BASIC TRAINING POSTURE

The posture you adopt when doing an exercise determines everything, actually. With good posture, you get the most out of the exercise; with with poor posture, you harm your body. Therefore, pay extra attention to that perfect neutral position and the imprint position you can take if neutral is too hard for you!

There are two basic postures when training:

1. The neutral position of your spine. You almost always use it when lying, standing, or sitting.
2. The imprint position. You use this when the exercise is too hard to do from the neutral position. See it as a reserve position.

# Neutral Position

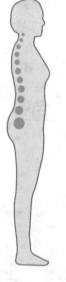

This is what your spine looks like in a neutral position:

You can see the natural S shape. But that S shape is very subtle, and you shouldn't confuse the curves with a hollow or rounded back. You should not have a hollow or rounded back in a neutral posture. These natural curves function as a shock absorber when you stand, jump, run, or simply walk around. Not only that, but in a neutral position, your muscles don't need to work as hard to keep you nice and upright and to get you moving.

You will notice that during the program we tell you a hundred times to pay attention to your neutral posture. There is a good reason for that because, without a neutral posture, you often do more harm than good. And take note: you should adopt a neutral posture ALWAYS—when sitting, lifting, squatting, lying down, cycling, on the toilet, and so on.

## This Is How You Find Your Spine's Neutral Posture

Lie down on the ground with your legs pulled up, with your feet hip-width apart and flat on the floor. If you are lying correctly, there will be two spots where your spine doesn't touch the floor: your neck and your lower back. Imagine you were to put a cup of coffee on your belly. If you are lying correctly, the coffee wouldn't spill. If you were to lie down with a hollow back, the coffee would spill over toward your pelvic bone. If you were to lie with a rounded back, the coffee would run toward your belly button. Neither is good; you want your coffee to stay in your cup. In other words, your hip bones and pelvic bone should be at the same height.

To check that you are lying in a good neutral posture, place your two thumbs and two index fingers against each other to make a triangle. Now place your fingers on your pelvic bone and your thumbs on your hips. Your hands should be parallel to the floor.

### Lying, Leaning Forward, Sitting, and Standing: Almost Always Your Neutral Posture

Your spine should always be in a neutral position, whether you are lying down, leaning forward, sitting, or standing. That is particularly difficult when you are lying down; therefore, pay extra attention to your spinal column. Before each exercise, check that you are in a neutral position. Do it again halfway through the exercise. If the exercise starts getting tough, there's a good chance you will use strength from elsewhere and forget your neutral posture.

# Imprint Position

It can be difficult to maintain a neutral position sometimes. If that's the case, you can switch to the "imprint" position. This position maintains and protects the stability of your pelvis and your lower back. It could be advisable for you to use the imprint position if you have weak abdominal muscles. In this position, it is easier to maintain the connection with your abdominal muscles and, at the same time, you strengthen your abdominal muscles so that you will eventually be able to do the exercises in your neutral posture.

### This is how you find your spine's imprint position

Lie down on the floor, knees pulled up, feet on the floor hip-width apart. Inhale gently while lying still and, as you exhale, bring your pelvic bone upward toward your belly button. Your lower back is now extended, lying on the mat, and is supported by your deepest abdominal muscles.

# PHASE 1:
# BACK

Y ou are still recuperating from the birth, you haven't even had the chance to admire your baby from head to toe yet, and your body is already switching to the first phase of our program. You can see the first phase, "Back," both literally as well as figuratively.

Your body is going back to caring for you alone. It must build up its cycle, rebalance its hormones, and reduce the size of your womb, and you need to recover from any direct trauma, such as a tear of incision or even a cesarean section. Your body will start making cells to close the wound, and the skin, connective tissue, and the muscles will go back to the condition they were in before the birth.

In the "Back" phase, you symbolically take a step back. Your body and your mind need time to come to terms with everything and to enjoy these wonderful first weeks together. These are emotional weeks, weeks you will never forget, and they have an enormous impact on the start of a new life.

This is what you can expect in this phase:
- Practical matters: postpartum health issues
- Practical matters: caring for lacerations
- Practical matters: caring for and recovering from a cesarean section
- Experts: the best "Back" tips from the experts

## YOUR LIFE IS NOW IN FAST-FORWARD, YOUR BODY STARTS WITH "BACK."

If you gave birth some time ago and you want to start the BTY recovery program, then you can skip to the "You" Phase (see page 218).

Fill in your starting data on page 291 before starting a new phase. It will give you an insight into your progress.

# Postpartum Health Issues

The first week is all about enjoying your baby, of course. But your body is also recovering from the amazing performance it has just accomplished. Here are the most common health issues after childbirth and what you can do to relieve the symptoms.

**HEMORRHOIDS:** Hemorrhoids are blood vessels in and around the anus that have swollen too much. They could feel itchy or give you a burning sensation, and you could even lose blood. One of the ways you get hemorrhoids is from pushing too hard, which you had to do during labor. Drinking plenty of water can help, as can eating fiber-rich foods to prevent constipation and not pushing when you go to the bathroom. Keep the hemorrhoids clean!

**UTERINE CRAMPS (POSTPARTUM CONTRACTIONS):** Almost straight after the birth, your uterus starts contracting. And as soon as you feel it, you will understand why we use the word *contraction*. These cramps are also called postpartum contractions. There is a wound where the placenta was attached to the womb. The more and better the uterus contracts, the quicker the wound closes. You will often notice you have more cramps when breastfeeding or when you hear your baby cry and your body reacts automatically with the let-down reflex. The let-down reflex is caused by the hormone oxytocin. It ensures the muscles around the milk ducts contract. But that hormone also causes the uterus to contract. Warm compresses and light massages can help (but, of course, not if you have had a cesarean section). Place your child on the breast frequently and go to the bathroom regularly. Your uterus can contract better with an empty bladder.

**SORE PELVIC FLOOR:** After childbirth, the tissue of the vagina, the anus, and the perineum (region between the vagina and anus) could be swollen or sore. It helps to air it! Lying down on a hydrophilic mat with a naked butt every so often can do wonders. A cushion may appear to bring relief, but it actually lengthens the healing process. Try to sit on a firm surface and upright. Push out the fluid, as it were. Pay attention to your posture; sitting or lying in the wrong position can cause other issues.

**PAINFUL BREASTS (ENGORGEMENT):** When breastfeeding is underway, your breasts will grow rapidly. They get rounder than round, and you feel it, too. Engorgement can even be painful. What often helps is to feed your baby frequently and make sure they drink until your breast is empty. A hot shower can also offer relief, and bruised, chilled cabbage leaves can also work wonders. Most women feel the engorgement between three to five days after childbirth, but it could also flare up a few days after that.

**LOSING FLUIDS (FREQUENT URINATION AND [NIGHT] SWEATS):** You hold on to extra fluid when you are pregnant, and you need to lose that now. You will urinate more often, but also you lose fluid through sweating. And that sweating mainly flares up at night. You could even wake up drenched in sweat. It helps to drink plenty of water. You can also put a clean T-shirt next to your bed so that, if you wake up in the night and are cold from lying in that first wet shirt, you have a dry one handy to change into.

**BLOOD LOSS:** You will lose a lot of blood in those first days, and mainly on the first day. You will see clots in the blood, and they can be quite big. If you don't need to change your maternity pads more frequently than every 30 minutes, you feel fine, and don't have a temperature, then it's perfectly normal. What helps is time . . . your womb simply needs time to heal. The worst bleeding will be over after the first week after childbirth. In the weeks after, it will start looking more like the bleeding you are used to seeing during your period. You can't have sex until you have stopped bleeding completely, which means the wound has healed.

**HAIR LOSS:** Suddenly, it seems like all your hair is falling out. Your brush is filled with hair after brushing. Don't worry; you are not going bald. You held on to extra hair during your pregnancy and now it's over, so you lose all that extra hair.

**CRYING/BABY BLUES:** The whole postpartum period is not one pink fluffy cloud. Over three-quarters of women suffer from baby blues to a greater or lesser degree. You are suddenly sad, need to cry, feel negative or depressing feelings, and you have no idea why. Guess what? It's those hormones. The sudden drop in progesterone can cause heavy emotions. It can help to know that you are not the issue—it's just your hormones and it will pass by itself. And a hug. That always helps.

# Lacerations, Incisions, and Care

During the delivery, something enormous had to come out of what is normally a tiny hole. You could have torn (laceration) or your physician may have made an incision (episiotomy). These are recommended ways to care for wounds.

## Recovering from a Tear or Incision

- In most cases, the stitches will fall out by themselves (dissolvable stitches) around day 10.
- Urine can be painful on the open wound. Urinate under the shower with the jet aimed at your vagina. It will wash away the stinging urine.
- Don't rub: dab!
- You have an open wound, so hygiene is important. You don't want to get an infection.
- Wounds heal quicker when exposed to the open air. Lie on a maternity mat to catch any blood you lose (very normal) and regularly air your vagina.
- Cooling can help. You can wrap an icepack in a towel and hold it against your vagina.
- Keep the scar supple by massaging it. You can do that once the physician declares the wound has "healed" and by using a special technique (see page 178).

## Recovering from a Cesarean Section

If you were advised against a vaginal birth, you would have had a cesarean section. And no matter how good and quick this method is, it is still abdominal surgery. Your skin was cut, and your muscles moved to the sides, which means you will need longer to recover than after a vaginal birth. This is what you can expect, and these are some helpful tips for you to recover as quickly and healthily as possible:

- After a cesarean section, you will probably stay in hospital for two to five days.
- The anesthesia or epidural could make you feel shaky or nauseous.
- Rest is particularly important, but you should try and walk a little very day. Keep moving!
- In most cases, you can urinate normally when the bladder catheter has been removed one day after childbirth.
- Don't lift anything heavier than your baby.

- The wound will close after three weeks, and the scar will start to disappear about six months after childbirth. You could have a dull sensation for weeks to months around the skin where the incision was made.
- You could feel more tired than usual for up to three to four months.
- Don't do abdominal muscle exercises until your physician says you can.
- Avoid exercises and movements where you bend backward.
- You can start doing pelvic floor muscle exercises earlier!
- Keep your scar supple by massaging it. You can do that once the physician declares the wound has "healed" and by using a special technique (see page 178).

## "BACK" TIPS FROM THE EXPERTS

### DR. SHEILA DE LIZ, gynecologist, Wiesbaden, Germany

The first weeks are all about surviving. No matter how well you prepared yourself, the wave of emotions will overwhelm you. Accept the situation for what it is and switch to survival mode. My best tips:

- **Let people help you.** If you have visitors coming, ask them to help. You don't have to play at being the perfect hostess right now. Ask them to make the tea or do that one little household chore that can't wait until any partner you have returns.
- **Order online.** Taking a trip to the store between feeds with a tiny baby and having to carry three bags of groceries is not a good idea right now. And why would you do that to yourself, your baby, your peace of mind, and your body when you can have your groceries delivered to your home?
- **Accept that things go at a different pace right now.** Not right now, thank you very much! Your biggest enemies right now are time pressure and setting the bar too high. Even if you don't shower for a few days . . . who cares?
- **Build a bond with your baby.** This is the most important thing right now. Make contact, be together, and enjoy it. If you are having trouble bonding, contact your physician immediately. There is a chance you are not producing specific substances. A lack of them could lead to postpartum depression.

## DR. MIRANDA GOËRTZ, psychologist, Arnhem, the Netherlands

As a mother, the way you experience the world is quite different compared to how your baby experiences the world. When you do something, you see it right away. Your baby reflects how you feel. Take a moment to think about that so that you can become aware of it. When you realize that your baby instantly picks up on your feelings, you have more reason to take care of yourself. When you feel comfortable in your own skin, your baby will feel comfortable in their own skin, too. If you feel out of balance, you should do something about it. It will be good for you and (therefore) for your baby, too. When you give yourself that balance, you give your baby that balance, too. *Food for thought!*

## BETÜL BERTHOLD, former mental health counselor and mother, Frankfurt, Germany

Betül has been working for years with pregnant women and women who have just given birth. She is known for her caring support, and one of the main things she does it teach women how they can help themselves get Back To You in the best possible way. The following are her tips.

- **Eat healthily.** It seems needless to say, but it is so important. Nutrients really are your best friend during your recovery. Your body needs the vitamins, minerals, and fiber, and your mind needs the energy you get from healthy food. Fast food is really bad for your body right now. You can see what your body really needs at the moment on page 74.
- **Sleep when your baby sleeps.** You really need your rest, and let's be honest, you don't get your eight hours a night. Make a point of it: sleep when baby sleeps. And if that doesn't work, just lie down and rest.
- **Write a letter to yourself.** Describe the genuine admiration you have for what you are doing. It sounds crazy, but giving yourself such a compliment really works wonders. Think about all the things you are doing well. When you read it later, it will make you feel good about yourself.
- **Try meditation.** You can meditate fairly easily and without a lot of fuss even if you are not used to it. There are apps available that have nice short stories and lovely sounds to listen to. Concentrate on the

sound, forget everything else, and you'll notice how your body and mind relax.

- **Relax using breathing techniques.** Recognize the first signs of physical tension. You often notice signs of stress through cramping in the shoulders, jaw, or other place on your face or in your neck. Everyone experiences stress on a different place of the body. As soon as you know your body's stress point, start doing breathing exercises. Sit down quietly and inhale deeply, visualize how the tense spot relaxes, and then exhale for longer than you inhaled. Practice this regularly. The more you do it, the easier it will become and the greater the effect will be.

- **Drink plenty.** Water is your set go-to now. It helps rebalance your hormones and hydrates your body, which is something you desperately need right now, especially if you are breastfeeding.

- **Take a few minutes for yourself every day.** Think about the wonderful changes you see in yourself. Try to embrace the flood of emotions; they may not always be positive, but they are part of it. Try to turn any negative feelings into positive strengths (e.g., you could feel overwhelmed, but you are getting on with it and you should be proud of that!).

- **Enjoy a couple minutes of silence every day.** I am a great believer in silence. With everything that's going on around you, it's wonderful to enjoy the silence for a few minutes every day. Silence calms and energizes you at the same time.

- **Don't pass baby from one person to the next.** In large families in particular, you often see that everyone comes to visit at the same time, and everyone wants to hold baby. If that's okay with you, go for it, but don't hold back your feelings. If you don't want it, say so. It will give you a sense of calm. And your baby, too.

- **Don't lose your identity as a woman.** Spoil yourself that little extra during these weeks, and actually for the rest of your life as a mother. Just because you are a mother, you shouldn't forget yourself. You are worth it and deserve it!

## ANN-MARLENE HENNING, sex and relationship therapist, Hamburg, Germany

- **Do your homework!** In the "Back" phase, it is important to learn about yourself, your body, and the new "you." That knowledge will calm your entire system. Get to know your body and feel your body. Grab a mirror and look at your whole body; therefore, also your vulva. Do it right away, in fact. Make contact with your body and remember, whatever you feel is okay!

- **Be aware that your breasts and uterus are neurologically connected.** When you are breastfeeding, your womb can spasm as your baby drinks from your breasts. This is a perfectly normal connection, and it enables your womb to return to its former size. That connection could feel like "lust." But know that the feeling is purely the (neurophysiological and evolutionary) connection between the uterus and breast.

# Training in the "Back" Phase

For women who have just given birth, we start slowly, but these gentle conscious exercises are the ones that will help you right now. Women who gave birth a while ago can skip Block 1 (Weeks 1–3). You can start with Block 2 straight away. You do that for one week instead of three. Therefore, you start your second week with the "To" phase right away. It is good to do the first week, in any case, because it makes you aware of your pelvic floor in relation to the rest of your body and your breathing. It will be easy for you, but it is a good start for anyone who has brought a beautiful new life into the world.

## For This Phase, You Will Need:

- Chair

## Your Daily BTY Kegel Exercises

Start with tensing for one second and then relaxing for one second. It's not long, but it's good to regain a grip on the muscles and to enable your brain to feel the connection with this muscle. During these weeks, take the time to come to grips with this tensing and relaxing principle by making this pumping-like action. In the second block of the "Back" phase, you increase it to three seconds.

## Do These Things Daily

- BTY Kegel exercises (see page 139)
- Walking
- Stretching, activating, and rolling (see page 127)

What the icons mean:

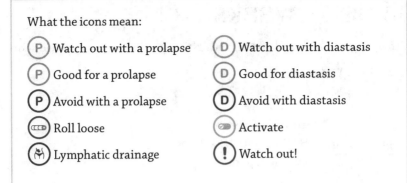

(P) Watch out with a prolapse    (D) Watch out with diastasis

(P) Good for a prolapse    (D) Good for diastasis

(P) Avoid with a prolapse    (D) Avoid with diastasis

Roll loose    Activate

Lymphatic drainage    (!) Watch out!

# BLOCK 1: WEEKS 1–3

Stretching your body and making the first connection with your pelvic floor.

▶ Open your app and join in with the training

**Pre-Workout**

**10 x XL Breath**
**BTY Kegel:** 10 x 1 sec
**Warm-Up:** none

## WORKOUT

**Neck Stretches**

| | WEEK 1 | ⬤ ⬤ ⬤ |
| --- | --- | --- |
| | WEEK 2 | ⬤ ⬤ ⬤ |
| | WEEK 3 | ⬤ ⬤ ⬤ |

**Calf Stretches**

| | WEEK 1 | ⬤ ⬤ ⬤ |
| --- | --- | --- |
| | WEEK 2 | ⬤ ⬤ ⬤ |
| | WEEK 3 | ⬤ ⬤ ⬤ |

**Brain–Pelvic Floor Connection**
**(LYING DOWN)**

| | WEEK 1 | ⬤ ⬤ ⬤ |
| --- | --- | --- |
| | WEEK 2 | ⬤ ⬤ ⬤ |
| | WEEK 3 | ⬤ ⬤ ⬤ |

## Chest and Side Body Stretches

WEEK 1
WEEK 2
WEEK 3

## Shoulder Stretches

WEEK 1
WEEK 2
WEEK 3

## Reverse Fly (SITTING)

Chest

Upper back
& shoulders

WEEK 1
WEEK 2
WEEK 3

## Mini (CHAIR) Squat  (P)

Thighs, buttocks
& calves

Legs & buttocks

WEEK 1
WEEK 2
WEEK 3

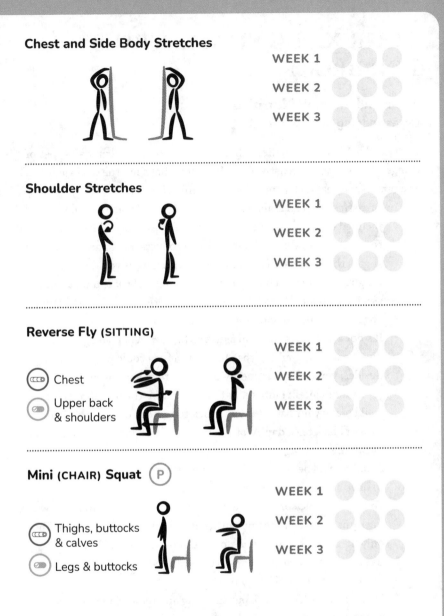

**Cool Down:** 15-minute walk

Circle: o = roll loose / **o** = activate
Add an arrow where you need to pay attention to
your neutral posture

# YOUR XL FUNDAMENTALS FOR BLOCK 1

## XL Fundamental: Nutrition
### Breastfeeding and your food

You're lucky. We used to believe that you couldn't eat or drink all types of things when you were breastfeeding. We know that's not the case anymore. You can actually eat and drink almost anything, but . . .

1. Breastfeeding can demand a lot of energy, and you might be inclined to eat more. It can do no harm to eat a little bit more (of course, we are talking about healthy products, not snacks and sugars that give a quick energy boost). As long as you don't gain weight, you are not consuming too much. A rule of thumb is that you burn about 300 to 500 additional calories when breastfeeding. That is comparable to one small meal.
2. It's not a good idea to go on a diet right now. When you go on a diet, your body could release toxins that you could pass on to baby. Besides, you need your energy to take care of your baby.
3. Limit your caffeine intake. Caffeine gets into the breast milk and could make your baby restless. Stick to one cup of coffee and two cups of black tea a day. Avoid energy drinks that are filled with lots of caffeine and sugar.
4. Avoid alcohol because it also gets into the breast milk. If you want to have a glass, do so right after feeding.
5. You can eat spicy or hot food, but if your infant seems to be showing signs of food allergy or sensitivity, check with your doctor. The only herbs you should avoid now are aloe, senna, and kava.
6. Eat fatty fish no more than twice a week because it could contain harmful dioxins and heavy metals.
7. It may be needless to say, but smoking and recreational drugs are not good for you or your baby, of course.

**DONE?   YES ●   NO ●**

## XL Fundamental: Rest and Relaxation
### Total relaxation

Sit or lie down with your baby. When you are both sitting comfortably against each other, relax your body completely. Start with your feet, then your lower legs, your knees, and your thighs. Feel each body part and work your way up until you feel that even your earlobes are relaxed. Be aware of what you are doing. Visualize it. You'll notice your baby will automatically take over this relaxed state. Your baby reacts to your body language like no other and will physically assume the calmness.

DONE? YES ◯ NO ◯

## XL Fundamental: Posture and Breathing
### Don't overstretch your thumbs

A mom thumb . . . ever heard of it? Many parents (and not only moms!) suffer from painful thumbs at a certain point. There is a simple reason for it: if you stretch your thumbs excessively each time you pick up your baby, you could develop symptoms. Your thumbs will feel tense and painful even when you are not using them. During these weeks, make a point of not overstretching your thumbs, instead clamping them when you pick up baby. Or even better for you and your baby, don't pick up your child under the armpits as often, but use one hand to support their shoulder and back. And place your other hand underneath, right along the spine.

DONE? YES ◯ NO ◯

## XL Fundamental: Exercise and Training
### Alternate lifting from left and right

It is not good for your body to lift or put down something from a lopsided position. But it's not always possible to lift and put down your baby straight ahead of you; consider this when putting baby in the crib or playpen. One thing that can help is to alternate. For one week, place baby in their crib while leaning from the left, and then the next week, move the crib a little so you can get to them from the other side.

DONE? YES ◯ NO ◯

**NOTES:**

_____

_____

_____

_____

# DIARY: BLOCK 1

Time for self-analysis. Fill in after you complete Block 1.

## Nutrition

| *How are you getting on with:* | VERY WELL | GOOD | COULD BE BETTER | BADLY |
|---|---|---|---|---|
| Eating healthy food? | ○ | ○ | ○ | ○ |
| Balancing protein, fat, and carbohydrates? | ○ | ○ | ○ | ○ |
| Drinking 1.5 liters of water daily? | ○ | ○ | ○ | ○ |
| Spreading out eating throughout the day? | ○ | ○ | ○ | ○ |

## Rest and Relaxation

*How are you getting on with:*          AARGH                    GOOD

Your inner levels of rest?

The demands you place on yourself?

Letting others help you?

Maintaining an overview?

Getting enough sleep?

## Posture and Breathing

| *Do you pay attention to:* | YES | REGULARLY | NOT ENOUGH | NO |
|---|---|---|---|---|
| Maintaining a good neutral posture all day? | ○ | ○ | ○ | ○ |
| Good posture when lifting your baby? | ○ | ○ | ○ | ○ |
| Good XL Breathing? | ○ | ○ | ○ | ○ |
| Using XL Breath when lifting? | ○ | ○ | ○ | ○ |

## Exercise and Training

| | YES | REGULARLY | NOT ENOUGH | NO |
|---|---|---|---|---|
| Do you notice progress during the training sessions? | ○ | ○ | ○ | ○ |

How many steps do you manage to do a day?

0 steps                              Minimum goal: 10,000                    15,000

## General Questions

*How are you getting on with:*    **AARGH**                    **GOOD**

Your hormones?

The bond with your child?

Your relationship?

Intimate contact?

Social life?

Work?

## Pelvic Floor Muscles and Abdominal Muscle Checkup

*How often do you do the:*    **NEVER**                    **EVERY DAY**

BTY Kegel?

XL Breath?

**Reminder:** Before starting the next block, check yourself for knots in your pelvic floor muscles (see page 143). If you find any, get rid of them first before continuing with your daily BTY Kegel exercises!

|  | YES | A LITTLE | NO |
|---|---|---|---|
| Are you still suffering from a large diastasis? | ○ | ○ | ○ |
| Are you still suffering from a prolapse? | ○ | ○ | ○ |
| Do you notice any progress in your pelvic floor muscles? | ○ | ○ | ○ |

## Based on My Self-Analysis:

These are the goals for the following block:

_____

_____

_____

This is how I am going to do that:

_____

_____

_____

# BLOCK 2: WEEKS 4–6

This is how you make (and maintain) the connection with your pelvic floor and your pelvic floor maintains that connection with the rest of your powerhouse.

▶ Open your app and join in with the training

**Pre-Workout**

**10 x XL Breath**
**BTY Kegel:** 10 x 3 sec (or 2 or 1 if you can't manage 3 seconds)
**Warm-Up:** none

## WORKOUT

**PF Lift 1** (P) (☺)

WEEK 1 ● ● ●
WEEK 2 ● ● ●

**PF Lift 2** (P) (D)

WEEK 3 ● ● ●

**Brain–Pelvic Floor Connection** (☺)
(LYING DOWN)

WEEK 1 ● ● ●
WEEK 2 ● ● ●
WEEK 3 ● ● ●

**Heel Slide** (☺)

WEEK 1 ● ● ●
WEEK 2 ● ● ●
WEEK 3 ● ● ●

**Namaste**

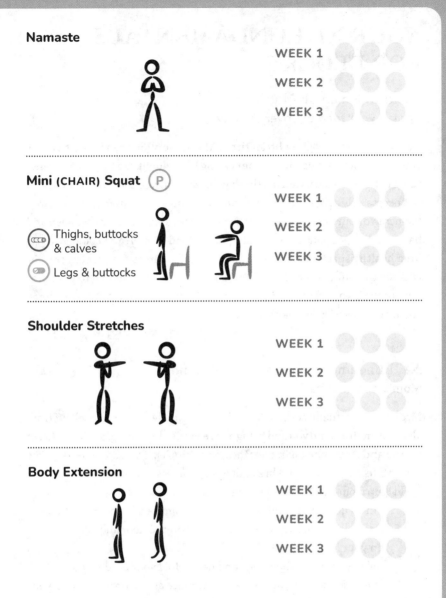

| | | | |
|---|---|---|---|
| WEEK 1 | ● | ● | ● |
| WEEK 2 | ● | ● | ● |
| WEEK 3 | ● | ● | ● |

**Mini (CHAIR) Squat** (P)

Thighs, buttocks & calves

Legs & buttocks

| | | | |
|---|---|---|---|
| WEEK 1 | ● | ● | ● |
| WEEK 2 | ● | ● | ● |
| WEEK 3 | ● | ● | ● |

**Shoulder Stretches**

| | | | |
|---|---|---|---|
| WEEK 1 | ● | ● | ● |
| WEEK 2 | ● | ● | ● |
| WEEK 3 | ● | ● | ● |

**Body Extension**

| | | | |
|---|---|---|---|
| WEEK 1 | ● | ● | ● |
| WEEK 2 | ● | ● | ● |
| WEEK 3 | ● | ● | ● |

**Cool Down:** 15-minute walk

Circle: O = roll loose / O = activate
Add an arrow where you need to pay attention to
your neutral posture

# YOUR XL FUNDAMENTALS FOR BLOCK 2

## XL Fundamental: Nutrition
**Spread your food out over the day**

Do you feel listless? Or (a little) tired? The amount of sleep you get affects your energy levels, but so does your eating behavior. It can help to eat something in between meals during the day. Spread out your food over the day. It's not necessarily about eating more but spreading it out differently. See what happens to your energy levels when you eat two small meals in between and have smaller portions for breakfast, lunch, and dinner. You could also opt for a healthy snack instead of a small meal. Examples are a wheat cracker with avocado (filled with good fats!), a hard-boiled egg (adding to your protein intake is good for muscle recovery), slaw (fiber for your bowels), or some yogurt with berries (probiotic bomb).

DONE?   YES ◯   NO ◯

## XL Fundamental: Rest and Relaxation
**Mom's mini meditation**

Meditation is actually nothing more than completely closing yourself off from all the stimuli around you and being aware of your breathing. See it as a Reset button and Pause button in one. The great thing is, if you do this every day, you will feel very calm and break down the stress hormones in your body. Build it up from 3 to 10 minutes a day.

1. Find a quiet place and sit upright in a comfortable position. For example, sit on a chair with your feet on the floor and your hands on your legs.
2. Relax your back, shoulders, and neck. Hold your head straight ahead. Make sure you also relax your face as you breathe. Relax your jaw, your cheeks, and your eyes. Your tongue is also in a relaxed position in your mouth, with the point just behind your teeth.
3. Now concentrate on your breathing. Gently breathe in and out, and be aware of your breathing. Try to close yourself off from the sounds and other impressions from outside or the thoughts that pop into your head. If you get lost in your thoughts, it's okay; just try to shift your focus back to your breathing.

DONE?   YES ◯   NO ◯

## XL Fundamental: Posture and Breathing
### Check your mirror

This week, check yourself in a mirror more frequently as you walk past one or in a window with a good reflection. Are you standing straight? Are your shoulders nicely down and back? And . . . are your eyes pointed to the horizon rather than down? Of course, you can't walk with a perfect posture all day, but be aware of it and try, as often as you can, to keep your back straight, tense your belly a little (don't let it hang), chin up, and shoulders back and down.

**DONE?   YES ◯   NO ◯**

## XL Fundamental: Exercise and Training
### Do: use stickers

Stick small red stickers at five locations around your house at places you often go: the bathroom, by the changing table, by the faucet, etc. Each time you see a sticker, take a moment to take three to five deep and gentle breaths while concentrating on your pelvic floor. Feel how it responds to your breathing. Try to make three inhalations "longer" and "lift" your pelvic floor when exhaling. Your belly will also pull inward. It feels like you are zipping up a really tight zipper from your pelvic bone to just below your belly button. This is a calming exercise (it's a sort of mindfulness exercise) that teaches your brain to make a connection with your breathing, your pelvic floor, your abdominal and back muscles. The more often you do this, the better the parts of your powerhouse will work in unison.

**DONE?   YES ◯   NO ◯**

### NOTES:

_____

_____

_____

_____

_____

# DIARY: BLOCK 2

Time for self-analysis. Fill in after you complete Block 2.

## Nutrition

| *How are you getting on with:* | VERY WELL | GOOD | COULD BE BETTER | BADLY |
|---|---|---|---|---|
| Eating healthy food? | ○ | ○ | ○ | ○ |
| Balancing protein, fat, and carbohydrates? | ○ | ○ | ○ | ○ |
| Drinking 1.5 liters of water daily? | ○ | ○ | ○ | ○ |
| Spreading out eating throughout the day? | ○ | ○ | ○ | ○ |

## Rest and Relaxation

| *How are you getting on with:* | AARGH | GOOD |
|---|---|---|
| Your inner levels of rest? | | |
| The demands you place on yourself? | | |
| Letting others help you? | | |
| Maintaining an overview? | | |
| Getting enough sleep? | | |

## Posture and Breathing

| *Do you pay attention to:* | YES | REGULARLY | NOT ENOUGH | NO |
|---|---|---|---|---|
| Maintaining a good neutral posture all day? | ○ | ○ | ○ | ○ |
| Good posture when lifting your baby? | ○ | ○ | ○ | ○ |
| Good XL Breathing? | ○ | ○ | ○ | ○ |
| Using XL Breath when lifting? | ○ | ○ | ○ | ○ |

## Exercise and Training

| | YES | REGULARLY | NOT ENOUGH | NO |
|---|---|---|---|---|
| Do you notice progress during the training sessions? | ○ | ○ | ○ | ○ |

How many steps do you manage to do a day?

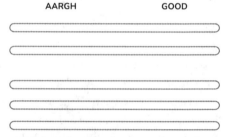

0 steps          Minimum goal: 10,000          15,000

## General Questions

*How are you getting on with:*    AARGH                     GOOD

Your hormones?

The bond with your child?

Your relationship?

Intimate contact?

Social life?

Work?

## Pelvic Floor Muscles and Abdominal Muscle Checkup

*How often do you do the:*    NEVER                    EVERY DAY

BTY Kegel?

XL Breath?

> **Reminder:** Before starting the next block, check yourself for knots in your pelvic floor muscles (see page 143). If you find any, get rid of them first before continuing with your daily BTY Kegel exercises!

|  | YES | A LITTLE | NO |
|---|---|---|---|
| Are you still suffering from a large diastasis? | ○ | ○ | ○ |
| Are you still suffering from a prolapse? | ○ | ○ | ○ |
| Do you notice any progress in your pelvic floor muscles? | ○ | ○ | ○ |

## Based on My Self-Analysis:

These are the goals for the following block:

_____

_____

This is how I am going to do that:

_____

_____

_____

# PHASE 2: TO

The first weeks have probably flown by. You have been bombarded with so many new impressions, which took some getting used to. In fact, you are probably still getting used to things. The first weeks, when you lived in a sort of cocoon or bubble, are over. You start working again, your social life starts up again, and your schedule is filling up again. You will increasingly need to move toward or "To" your normal life again.

This is the time for your checkup to see that any wounds have closed and that your uterus has recovered (it now weighs 2.1 ounces; it weighed 2.2 pounds at the end of the pregnancy!). From a medical perspective, the physician or midwife will give you the go-ahead so that you can go back "To" your normal life. You can have sex again, you can massage your scars to minimize any health issues, you can play sports again, and drive the car again if you had a cesarean section. Although you can do all these things again from a medical perspective, it doesn't mean it's easy to go back "To" normal life on an emotional level. That, too, could take some getting used to, and it takes time. And be aware, the brain doesn't like change. If you let undesirable habits sneak into your life now, it will be increasingly difficult to turn back the clock later. In this phase, be aware of how you want to approach your life and make that your new habit.

This is what you can expect in this phase:
- Practical matters: returning to work
- Practical matters: contraception
- Experts: helpful "To" tips
- Experts: massaging your scars

## YOU GRADUALLY PICK UP THE THREAD AGAIN AND GO "TO" THE WORLD OUTSIDE YOUR BUBBLE.

# Back to Work

One woman looks forward to it, another dreads going back to work. These practical tips will really make it easier to make the transition "To" your work life.

**TIME TO GET USED TO A CAREGIVER:** Your little baby will also go "To" a new phase in their young life. Whether you have chosen to use a babysitter, a daycare center, or or Grandma and Grandad to look after baby, you and your baby will both need to get used to the new situation. Do a few practice runs before going back to work. If you find it hard to cope, you can collect baby right away. It takes time to get used to it all, so give yourself and your baby that time.

**VISIT YOUR WORKPLACE:** A few days before you start working again, go to your workplace with your baby. Your colleagues will get to see your baby and have a picture in their head when you tell them 101 lovely stories later on. And a major bonus: you will get a taste of the atmosphere at work again. You will hear the latest gossip and how things are going, and it won't be such a shock to your system on your first working day back.

**AGREE WHO DOES WHAT:** For those with a partner, it's time to agree how the chores will be divided up between you. Who does what in the house? Who will leave work on which day if the caregiver calls to say that baby is sick, for instance? Making agreements is good for your relationship. Many relationships fall apart because women take on too much and then blame the man afterward because they were not proactive enough in family life. Really, making agreements gives a sense of calm.

**PREPARATIONS:** The more you prepare, the easier your day will start and end. Get as many things ready in the evening as you can. So, lay out your clothes, your baby's clothes, and pack your bag and your baby's bag. Set the breakfast table, if necessary. The morning rush hour is terribly busy with a baby, and anything you can do in the evening will make all the difference. Plan your menu for the week and do your grocery shopping on the weekend for the whole week. It will save you time every day. And besides that, you'll be in no mood to go to the grocery store with a baby in tow at the end of the working day.

**START IN THE MIDDLE OF THE WEEK:** It would seem logical to go back to work on a Monday, but experience has shown that it's often much better to start halfway through the week. Working half a week makes it easier for you and your baby to get used to the new situation.

# Contraception after Childbirth

Theoretically, you can get pregnant again right after childbirth. It usually takes a few months for your menstrual cycle to start up again, but because ovulation comes before the first period you can never be sure when you could get pregnant. Be safe rather than sorry and take precautions. You will probably have looked at the various kinds of contraception before now, but you should keep a few other things in mind with your postpartum body.

# "TO" TIPS FROM THE EXPERTS

## DR. JOLENE BRIGHTEN, naturopathic doctor, biochemist, and an expert in female hormones, Seattle, USA

It's clear that all contraception has the same effect, but a postpartum body can react differently, and you have to consider other circumstances and risks. We don't know enough about all the effects of certain birth control on our recovering body simply because there has not been enough conclusive research and the existing studies often contradict each other.

- **Hormonal contraception: Hormones affect you in all sorts of ways and not only your body.** In fact, many hormones, such as the pill, influence your brain. It changes hormone production in your brain, which influences your ovulation. That's pretty heavy if you think about it, and especially now, when all your hormones are upside down anyway.

    **There could be a possible link between developing (postpartum) depression and using hormonal contraception.** Although many studies are contradictory, we know there could be a link between using hormonal contraception and depression. It is notable that some data indicates that IUDs containing only progesterone cause the highest risk of mood disorders.

- **The pill: You have an increased risk of developing blood clots after childbirth.** The pill itself increases your risk of blood clots. By taking the pill, especially in the first months, you could increase the risk of blood clots even further.

- **Progestogen-only pill (mini pill): As the name suggests, this pill doesn't contain estrogen, and it is generally the first thing that physicians recommend to women after childbirth.** It is less effective than other pills at preventing pregnancy, but it could be a better choice because of the lower risk of clots.

- **Birth control shot (progestin): The birth control shot is an injectable progestin that works for three months.** There is also a potential link between this hormonal contraception and postpartum depression. Currently, there isn't any substantial proof that it contributes to postpartum depresison, but a lack of evidence doesn't exclude it. And forewarned is forearmed.

- **Intrauterine device (IUD): If you choose to use an IUD, you should wait at least six weeks until your womb has returned to its nor-

**mal size.** Women who had a preterm prelabor rupture of the membranes, who have an inflammation of the uterine lining, or who are still bleeding are advised against getting an IUD after childbirth. If you are breastfeeding, there is a slightly higher risk of perforation when the IUD is inserted.

- **Condoms: Condoms are completely safe during the postpartum period.** The downside is the "fiddling around"; the big plus is that no physical procedure is involved. You don't have a device inserted in your body for long periods of time, and you allow your hormones to find their place.

- **Tracking method (fertility awareness method [FAM]): This tracking method is effective, but many women find it hard to use in the postpartum period without the right support because their cycle is not as it was.** So, what data do you put in the app? If you are considering using the tracking method, you could ask your midwife or physician for some advice. You could even try to find a FAM coach. There are plenty of these coaches in the United States. You can also consult them via Skype. Don't forget that ovulation occurs before menstruation, so you shouldn't wait until your first period before taking steps to prevent pregnancy.

## DR. SHEILA DE LIZ, gynecologist, Wiesbaden, Germany

You are gradually coming out of your bubble and you are no longer simply surviving. You are rejoining life, and that could take some getting used to. Now is the time to recover your inner strength, to step into the outside world again, literally and figuratively. It's time to rejoin the carousel of life. My tips:

1. **Don't neglect yourself.** Be true to yourself.
2. **Now that you are a mother, stay yourself and even a stronger version of yourself.** That sounds vague, but it's an important tip. You may be a mother now, but you are still a woman, too. In this phase, the way you move "To" normal life, but now with a baby, will determine many things in the future. All too often, I see relationships fall apart when the children get older, and the cause may well have been the choices those women unconsciously made when they became a mother. No matter how difficult it is to find the balance between being a woman, partner, and mother, this phase of "To" is made to help you work on that. Your baby is your number one prior-

ity, of course, but forgetting or neglecting yourself is a danger zone you want to avoid. See also page 60.

3. **You can have sex again once your physician has checked your vagina.** It might not be on your mind at all or you may want to think about it first. And it makes perfect sense that you wouldn't want sex if you feel any pain or the skin opens and bleeds during penetration. And yet, you can do something about it! When you are breastfeeding, you don't have your regular cycle. It's nice you haven't gotten your period yet, but the downside is that your vagina could be dry. Compare it to an old sponge that has completely shrunk and shriveled up. It's not the nicest comparison to make with your vagina, but it's a clear one. That sponge must become nice and full, wet, and flexible again. One way to achieve that is by applying an estriol cream to the skin of the opening of the vagina. You will notice the difference within two to three weeks. Sex won't be painful, and you will be able to enjoy it again. The cream is only available by prescription; ask your physician about it!

4. **Do you think you have a prolapse?** If that's the case, have it checked by your physician or a pelvic therapist. Prolapses come in different degrees. A degree 1 or 2 prolapse, when the muscles aren't so stretched that you need surgical intervention, can be trained away with the BTY program. Degrees 3 and 4 need surgery, and if you can avoid that, do so. Those surgeries are drastic and can have lifelong consequences for your sex life, for example. Not all physicians consider the entire clitoris (which is much more than that little "bobble"; see page 48) and the neural pathways running through the vagina that play a role in sexual pleasure. Too often, the focus is on the urinary function. Therefore, if you have a degree 3 or 4 prolapse and really need surgery, make sure the surgeon will take your clitoris into consideration during the procedure. And don't forget: you can always ask for a different physician.

## ANN-MARLENE HENNING, sex and relationship therapist, Hamburg, Germany

This "To" phase is the phase to prevent any unwanted and undesirable patterns from slowly creeping into your mind. Those patterns will be there before you know it. Your brain doesn't like change; therefore, you will have to actively work on getting "To" the life you want to live.

1. **Don't only be the milking machine.** Make space for yourself, whether through work or going out with friends, take time for yourself, your person, and your body. And being with your baby doesn't count as time for yourself. Get someone else to look after your baby, even if it's only for two hours. You will feel human again and not only like a milking machine. And by taking this time, you will really miss being with your partner and baby.

2. **Be parents together.** It happens to many mothers and often without them realizing; they get overly enthusiastic about the baby. Pay attention to the little things between both partners. Make sure your partner "parents" just as much as you do. If the mother makes all the decisions and tells the co-mom or dad that they are doing things wrong all the time (even little things, such as which hat to put on baby), the mother is actually saying: "Stay out of it, this is my baby, and you are not part of it." That will affect your relationship, of course. Avoid that and be parents together. You will both feel valued and respected when you take the journey of parenthood together.

3. **Continue being partners, not only parents.** Remember that the brain easily falls back into old habits. You couldn't have sex during the "Back" phase, but now you can, so go for it! Enjoy parenthood together but also enjoy being together as a couple. In "Back," you learned to get to know your body (again); it's now time to start using that body again! That may be easier said than done for some, but really, with sex, it's use it or lose it. Sex is part of human life and is actually a very natural desire. But unlike hunger or sleep, sex isn't a drive. The difference is that you can survive without it. When you are really hungry, you eat. When you are really tired, you sleep. But you will have to do your best to get your sex life going. When you don't have sex, you want it less. The brain will reprogram itself and create a new habit. So, start experimenting with sex, enjoy your body, enjoy the sexual "you." Whether with your partner or alone, activate the sex part of your brain!

## DRS. MIRANDA GOËRTZ, psychologist, Arnhem, the Netherlands

We all know that childbirth affects your body and mind, but it is less well known that childbirth also influences your baby's self-confidence, the number of stimuli your baby can cope with, and the bond with you. After a birth trauma, it can be a good idea to help your baby find a better balance. When your baby is feeling balanced, motherhood will be easier and more pleasant because you will have a better bond between you both. Unfortunately, this is seen as very wishy-washy, but the impact of a birth trauma on self-confidence and a child's approach to life has not only been proven, but it can also even be physically measured in the brain.

1. There are specific methods to mimic your baby being born again; for example, by building a sort of tunnel or having baby reemerge "from the belly" by pulling them out from under a sweater. It is important to talk to your baby to let them know you understand what they have been through. You should do this fairly soon, but not right away in the "Back" phase. At that point, you are still in a sort of daze and surviving, and you aren't totally yourself, either. You can do it now in the "To" phase. Go to a psychologist who is specializes in bonding and birth traumas for advice so that you can do it yourself afterward.

2. A secure bond is even more important for babies who came into the world by cesarean section. When a baby cries, they feel a disbalance. That is often due to a massive number of stimuli. Therefore, comfort your child and let them know you are there for them. A baby who has had a birth trauma needs even more physical contact and closeness. It reinforces the feeling of "I am allowed to be here."

## MEDITATE TO GET CLOSER TO YOURSELF

Accept how you feel! Don't try to live up to all types of expectations. Stay as true to yourself as you can. But okay, at this stage, it's very normal if you have not totally found "yourself" yet. Meditation can be a great help. Meditation helps reduce stress levels, helps you keep less pleasant things at bay, and clears your head. You will get to know yourself better and it helps you set priorities.

1. Find a room where you can be alone and can have total peace and quiet for 10 minutes. You can also use essential oils at the same time, if you'd like to. Lavender is particularly good for relaxation. Myrrh is good at helping you clear your mind.

2. Sit in the lotus position or another comfortable position on a cushion. Make sure your back is straight, your chin slightly downward, and that you can draw a straight line from your crown to the sky. Squint your eyes. Concentrate on a point about 6 feet away.

3. Concentrate on your breathing. Inhale deeply through your nose three times and exhale deeply through your mouth. Leave your thoughts for what they are. Don't seek them out, but if they come, just be aware of them. Don't reject or judge them. Acknowledge them and leave them be. If you want to get rid of the thoughts that pop up, you can visualize them and "send them away." "Catch" your thoughts in a balloon and let it float into the air. Or put your thoughts on a leaf and let it drift away on the current of a river. After these visualizations, go back to your breathing.

4. In your mind, take a walk in a forest. Look at the forest around you and accept it for what it is.

5. Conclude by inhaling white light and exhaling a gray to brown light.

6. Don't get up straight away but take a moment to gather yourself. Do you have nice big smile on your face? If meditation is not for you, go for a walk in nature four times a week.

## MASSAGE YOUR SCARS. DO IT. DO IT. DO IT.

### LINDSEY VESTAL, MS, occupational therapist and pelvic floor expert, New York, USA

Scar tissue is tough, thick, and affects the entire area around the scar. The wound will have closed after a few weeks and the risk of infection will have passed, but you are not fully recovered yet and you may still notice the physical effects of the scar for a while if you wait for it to heal by itself.

It is much better to take charge of the situation as soon as your midwife or physician has declared your wound healed. It might sound a little strange, but it's really good to massage your scars and your entire perineum (the region between your anus and vagina).

1. Wash your hands. It may be obvious, but vaginal hygiene is particularly important.

2. Massage your scar and the surrounding area in a way that feels comfortable for you. Pay particular attention to the part that feels the toughest. Move the scar in that direction. When massaging, use an oil or cream that is safe for the vaginal tissue. For example, you could use a special perineum oil, coconut oil, or a product containing vitamin E.

3. If you also have damage inside your vagina, an external massage may not be enough and you will need to massage yourself internally, too (see page 143).

4. If you are really not in the mood for sex or anything closely related to it, remember that this type of massage is just like massaging any other body part. You would also apply a cream to any other scar and use the pressure of a massage to keep the tissue supple. Caring for your vagina in this way is nothing more than medical maintenance. But if you enjoy it, all the better. You can stick that feather in your cap.

5. And there is another benefit to perineum massages. Your pelvic floor plays a major role as a "pump" for your lymphatic system. By massaging your perineum, you activate the circulation, which helps your body get rid of excessive fluids from your system. Therefore, get over your embarrassment and start massaging.

## IF IT DIDN'T TURN OUT AS YOU IMAGINED AND YOU HAD A CESAREAN SECTION . . .

It's still a good idea to massage your perineum even if you gave birth by cesarean section. After all, it was under pressure for nine months. You won't have scars around your vagina, but you will on your belly. As soon as your physician says it's okay, you can get to work.

1. Lie down, and put your legs flat on the floor. Place your finger above your scar and make slow clockwise circles going from hip to hip. Then, follow the same line back but counterclockwise. Do the same again but underneath your scar.

2. Now, place your fingers on the same imaginary line above your scar and slowly move them up and down on the spot. Move your fingers over about ¾ inch and move them slowly up and down while exerting light pressure. Continue until you reach the other hip and follow the same line back. Do the same again, following an imaginary line under your scar.

3. Try to carefully pick up your scar bit by bit (roughly every half an inch): you pull up the skin a little.

4. Repeat steps 1 to 3, but with one leg pulled up. You will be able to go a little deeper.

5. Massage your scar for a couple of minutes three to five times per week.

**FACT:** If your scar tissue presses on your bladder and you have weak pelvic floor muscles, you could get symptoms of incontinence. This gives you even more reason to massage your scar and keep it supple.

## DR. SONIA BAHLANI, gynecologist, New York, USA

If you have issues with your bladder after a cesarean section but you've tested negative for a bladder infection, you might have an irritated bladder. Don't put up with it' go to your physician. The quicker you take these issues seriously, the better and easier they are to treat.

# Training in the "To" Phase

The first low-intensity workout can begin once your midwife or physician has said your wounds have healed properly and that you can start training again. That is generally after six to eight weeks.

But before you get started, you should answer these questions.

- Do you have a diastasis of over 0.87 inch (see self-test, page 261)? If so, pay attention to the icons next to the exercises.
- Do you have a prolapse (see self-test page, 264)? If so, pay attention to the icons next to the exercises.
- Do you have internal trigger points (see self-test, page 143)? If so, first get rid of the trigger points with an internal massage before continuing with your daily BTY Kegel exercises.

## For This Phase, You Will Need:

- Chair and cushion
- Towel
- Foam roller

## Your Daily BTY Kegel Exercises

In this phase, you build up your daily BTY Kegel exercises to five seconds. You should continue doing these three to four times a day, preferably for the rest of your life. Take note: only do the exercise for the length of time you can manage. This exercise is a blessing for life when done correctly, but you will harm your body if you do it incorrectly.

Fill in your starting data on page 291 before starting a new phase. It will give you an insight into your progress.

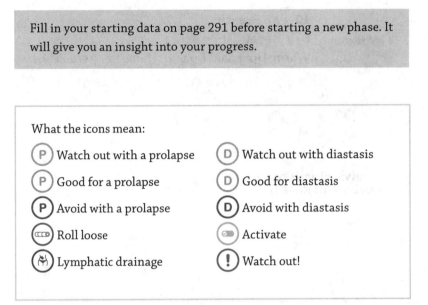

What the icons mean:

(P) Watch out with a prolapse

(P) Good for a prolapse

(P) Avoid with a prolapse

(ccco) Roll loose

(M) Lymphatic drainage

(D) Watch out with diastasis

(D) Good for diastasis

(D) Avoid with diastasis

(ca) Activate

(!) Watch out!

# BLOCK 3: WEEKS 7–9

You are going to start fixing your powerhouse and continue doing muscle lengthening, stretching exercises. You will work on the distribution of pressure by paying proper attention to your breathing.

▶ Open your app and join in with the training

**Pre-Workout**

**10 x XL Breath**
**BTY Kegel:** 10 x 4 sec
**Warm-Up:** Foam Rolling, Namaste, Aerobiclike

## WORKOUT

---

**Brain–Pelvic Floor Connection** (D)
**(ON HANDS AND KNEES)**

WEEK 1 ● ● ●
WEEK 2 ● ● ●
WEEK 3 ● ● ●

---

**Cat to Cow** (D)

⊙ Abdomen & lower back    ⊙ Lower back & upper back

WEEK 1 ● ● ●
WEEK 2 ● ● ●
WEEK 3 ● ● ●

---

**Heel Drop** (👤) (P)

⊙ Abdomen

WEEK 1 ● ● ●
WEEK 2 ● ● ●
WEEK 3 ● ● ●

---

## Adductor Ball

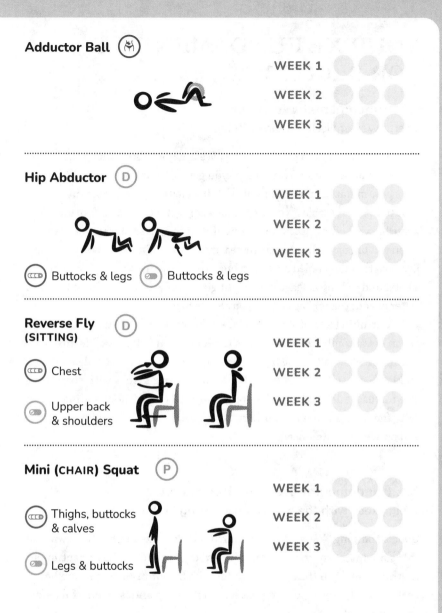

WEEK 1

WEEK 2

WEEK 3

## Hip Abductor (D)

WEEK 1

WEEK 2

WEEK 3

⬤ Buttocks & legs    ◯ Buttocks & legs

## Reverse Fly
(SITTING) (D)

⬤ Chest

◯ Upper back
& shoulders

WEEK 1

WEEK 2

WEEK 3

## Mini (CHAIR) Squat (P)

⬤ Thighs, buttocks
& calves

◯ Legs & buttocks

WEEK 1

WEEK 2

WEEK 3

**Cool Down:** Stretch neck, shoulders, legs

Circle: o = roll loose / o = activate
Add an arrow where you need to pay attention to
your neutral posture

# YOUR XL FUNDAMENTALS FOR BLOCK 3

## XL Fundamental: Nutrition
### The power of H$_2$O: balanced fluids

Fluid is essential for a good recovery. We are not talking about juices and coffee but about water. Water helps you get rid of any excessive fluids you have accumulated, and on top of that, it's particularly important to keep your fluid levels stable if you are breastfeeding. It can be nice to drink water while breastfeeding. Get into a habit of having a glass of water next to you when you breastfeed. Never drink tea or any other hot drink over your baby. Even tea that has cooled down can burn them. During these weeks, get into a habit of drinking at least six to eight glasses of water a day. Put a bottle of water in your diaper bag so that you always have water with you.

But drinking lots of water won't be effective if you consume a lot of salt. So, an extra combined challenge is to reduce your salt intake during these coming weeks. Salt is the biggest enemy for anyone who easily swells up and holds on to fluids anyway. Try to flavor your dishes with something else instead, such as herbs. Try to go three weeks without adding salt or salty flavorings (such as bouillon, soy sauce, or tamari), and you will see and notice the difference!

DONE?　YES ⬤　NO ⬤

## XL Fundamental: Rest and Relaxation
### Weightless with the most relaxing song in the world

Google the song "Weightless" by Marconi Union. Research has shown that this song instantly relaxes your mind and your body. It has a continuous rhythm of 60 bpm (beats per minute), which your brain waves and heartbeat instantly adjust to. It relaxes you right away and is wonderful before going to sleep!

DONE?　YES ⬤　NO ⬤

## XL Fundamental: Posture and Breathing
### Loosen your midriff

You need a mobilized midriff to do XL Breathing properly. As the space in your belly became increasingly limited during the pregnancy, you probably started chest breathing more, which you continue doing after childbirth. This could result in your midriff being tighter than usual. It is easy to loosen it. Stand straight and place your fingers just under the edge of your ribs. Push your fingers inward slightly and move them back and forth along the ribs. It will feel a little unnatural at first, but after doing it a few times, your midriff will feel more relaxed or looser.

**DONE?  YES       NO**

## XL Fundamental: Exercise and Training
### Treat your vagina to an oat bath

Yes, you read it right: put half a cup of oats in a hot bath, let it soak for 10 to 15 minutes, and it will be a real treat for your vagina. Oats have an anti-inflammatory effect; they reduce swelling and, as a bonus, they moisten the vagina.

**DONE?  YES       NO**

**NOTES:**

# DIARY: BLOCK 3

Time for self-analysis. Fill in after you complete Block 3.

## Nutrition

| How are you getting on with: | VERY WELL | GOOD | COULD BE BETTER | BADLY |
|---|---|---|---|---|
| Eating healthy food? | ○ | ○ | ○ | ○ |
| Balancing protein, fat, and carbohydrates? | ○ | ○ | ○ | ○ |
| Drinking 1.5 liters of water daily? | ○ | ○ | ○ | ○ |
| Spreading out eating throughout the day? | ○ | ○ | ○ | ○ |

## Rest and Relaxation

| How are you getting on with: | AARGH | GOOD |
|---|---|---|
| Your inner levels of rest? | | |
| The demands you place on yourself? | | |
| Letting others help you? | | |
| Maintaining an overview? | | |
| Getting enough sleep? | | |

## Posture and Breathing

| Do you pay attention to: | YES | REGULARLY | NOT ENOUGH | NO |
|---|---|---|---|---|
| Maintaining a good neutral posture all day? | ○ | ○ | ○ | ○ |
| Good posture when lifting your baby? | ○ | ○ | ○ | ○ |
| Good XL Breathing? | ○ | ○ | ○ | ○ |
| Using XL Breath when lifting? | ○ | ○ | ○ | ○ |

## Exercise and Training

| | YES | REGULARLY | NOT ENOUGH | NO |
|---|---|---|---|---|
| Do you notice progress during the training sessions? | ○ | ○ | ○ | ○ |

How many steps do you manage to do a day?

0 steps        Minimum goal: 10,000        15,000

## General Questions

*How are you getting on with:*

| | AARGH | GOOD |
|---|---|---|

Your hormones?

The bond with your child?

Your relationship?

Intimate contact?

Social life?

Work?

## Pelvic Floor Muscles and Abdominal Muscle Checkup

*How often do you do the:*

| | NEVER | EVERY DAY |
|---|---|---|

BTY Kegel?

XL Breath?

**Reminder:** Before starting the next block, check yourself for knots in your pelvic floor muscles (see page 143). If you find any, get rid of them first before continuing with your daily BTY Kegel exercises!

| | YES | A LITTLE | NO |
|---|---|---|---|
| Are you still suffering from a large diastasis? | ○ | ○ | ○ |
| Are you still suffering from a prolapse? | ○ | ○ | ○ |
| Do you notice any progress in your pelvic floor muscles? | ○ | ○ | ○ |

## Based on My Self-Analysis:

These are the goals for the following block:

_____

_____

This is how I am going to do that:

_____

_____

_____

# BLOCK 4: WEEKS 10–12

You will continue working on getting your abdominal muscles into shape, you will start doing light strength exercises, and you will do your first small and gentle rotations.

> ▶ Open your app and join in with the training

**Pre-Workout**
**10 x XL Breath**
**BTY Kegel:** 10 x 5 sec
**Warm-Up:** Foam Rolling and PF Lift 1 + 2

## WORKOUT

**Cat to Cow** (D)

Lower back & upper back    Abdomen & lower back

WEEK 1
WEEK 2
WEEK 3

**Heel Drop** (M) (P)

Abdomen

WEEK 1
WEEK 2
WEEK 3

**(MINI) Side Plank**

Abdomen

WEEK 1
WEEK 2
WEEK 3

## Pelvic Bridge Ⓟ

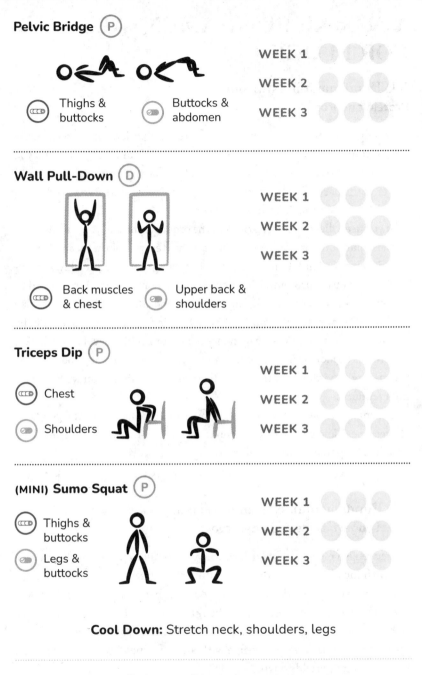

WEEK 1

WEEK 2

WEEK 3

Thighs & buttocks

Buttocks & abdomen

## Wall Pull-Down Ⓓ

WEEK 1

WEEK 2

WEEK 3

Back muscles & chest

Upper back & shoulders

## Triceps Dip Ⓟ

Chest

Shoulders

WEEK 1

WEEK 2

WEEK 3

## (MINI) Sumo Squat Ⓟ

Thighs & buttocks

Legs & buttocks

WEEK 1

WEEK 2

WEEK 3

**Cool Down:** Stretch neck, shoulders, legs

Circle: o = roll loose / o = activate
Add an arrow where you need to pay attention to
your neutral posture

# YOUR XL FUNDAMENTALS FOR BLOCK 4

## XL Fundamental: Nutrition
### Protein and Iron

Your body needs protein for muscle recovery during periods when you demand a lot of your muscles; therefore, just after childbirth and in the months you are training hard. You can find protein in fish, meat, dairy, and eggs. If you prefer plant-based foods, then legumes, vegetables, oats, nuts, and seeds contain the amino acids your body needs.

If you use a diet app to keep track of the products you eat, you will also find out how much protein you are consuming. Try to eat protein in the morning; it will make you feel full so that you will not get hungry again as quickly. In addition, when you eat protein-rich foods you burn more calories during the day.

Keep an eye on your iron levels during periods of recovery (whether due to childbirth or through training hard). Iron is found in animal products, mainly red meat, but green vegetables also contain high levels. The darker the green, the more iron. Your body can absorb iron better when you combine the meal with vitamin C and less well when you combine iron with milk or milk products.

During these weeks, try to combine protein, carbohydrates, and good fats in every meal, and pay extra attention to eating iron-rich products. Download an app to keep track of what you are eating and to figure out the right balance.

DONE?   YES ◯   NO ◯

## XL Fundamental: Rest and Relaxation
### Facial yoga: because you deserve it

There are also muscles in your face, and you should really train them every day with facial yoga. It's good for wrinkles and bags under the eyes. Bags under your eyes: pinch the skin under your eyes between your thumb, index, and middle fingers and gently pull the skin forward while closing your eyes tightly. Work from your nose to the outer corner of your eye. Frown lines: open your eyes as wide as possible without frowning! Do it 10 times while keeping your eyes wide open.

DONE?   YES ◯   NO ◯

## XL Fundamental: Posture and Breathing
### Check your XL Breathing

**LINDSEY VESTAL, MS,** occupational therapist and pelvic floor expert, New York, USA

Do you want to learn to do conscious 3D breathing? If so, then for five minutes every day, knot a TheraBand (an elastic gym band) around your waist at the bottom of your ribs and the part just under your ribs. The band will allow you to feel whether you are using your belly and your ribs.

**DONE? YES** ● **NO** ●

## XL Fundamental: Exercise and Training
### Use it or lose it

When it comes to your muscles, it's a case of use it or lose it. If you don't use them, they will get increasingly slack and you won't be as fit, and that has a negative impact on your healthy body composition. In short, during these coming weeks, keep telling yourself to keep up with the training. Think about the "use it or lose it" principle and make it your mantra.

**DONE? YES** ● **NO** ●

**DR. DORINE VAN RAVENSBERG,** human movement scientist, Voorthuizen, the Netherlands

You can also use a towel instead of a TheraBand. Hold it at the same height around your middle and hold the ends. When you inhale and allow the towel to move with the motion, you feel how your ribs move together and can "open." That is chest and flank breathing. If you don't move the towel with the motion, you will notice what your abdominal breathing does and how it does it. It will enable you to better understand how chest-flank breathing works and what it feels like.

**NOTES:**

_____

_____

_____

# DIARY: BLOCK 4

Time for self-analysis. Fill in after you complete Block 4.

## Nutrition

| *How are you getting on with:* | VERY WELL | GOOD | COULD BE BETTER | BADLY |
|---|---|---|---|---|
| Eating healthy food? | ○ | ○ | ○ | ○ |
| Balancing protein, fat, and carbohydrates? | ○ | ○ | ○ | ○ |
| Drinking 1.5 liters of water daily? | ○ | ○ | ○ | ○ |
| Spreading out eating throughout the day? | ○ | ○ | ○ | ○ |

## Rest and Relaxation

| *How are you getting on with:* | AARGH | GOOD |
|---|---|---|
| Your inner levels of rest? | | |
| The demands you place on yourself? | | |
| Letting others help you? | | |
| Maintaining an overview? | | |
| Getting enough sleep? | | |

## Posture and Breathing

| *Do you pay attention to:* | YES | REGULARLY | NOT ENOUGH | NO |
|---|---|---|---|---|
| Maintaining a good neutral posture all day? | ○ | ○ | ○ | ○ |
| Good posture when lifting your baby? | ○ | ○ | ○ | ○ |
| Good XL Breathing? | ○ | ○ | ○ | ○ |
| Using XL Breath when lifting? | ○ | ○ | ○ | ○ |

## Exercise and Training

| | YES | REGULARLY | NOT ENOUGH | NO |
|---|---|---|---|---|
| Do you notice progress during the training sessions? | ○ | ○ | ○ | ○ |

How many steps do you manage to do a day?

0 steps — Minimum goal: 10,000 — 15,000

## General Questions

*How are you getting on with:*

|  | AARGH | GOOD |
|---|---|---|
| Your hormones? | | |
| The bond with your child? | | |
| Your relationship? | | |
| Intimate contact? | | |
| Social life? | | |
| Work? | | |

## Pelvic Floor Muscles and Abdominal Muscle Checkup

*How often do you do the:*

|  | NEVER | EVERY DAY |
|---|---|---|
| BTY Kegel? | | |
| XL Breath? | | |

> **Reminder:** Before starting the next block, check yourself for knots in your pelvic floor muscles (see page 143). If you find any, get rid of them first before continuing with your daily BTY Kegel exercises!

|  | YES | A LITTLE | NO |
|---|---|---|---|
| Are you still suffering from a large diastasis? | ○ | ○ | ○ |
| Are you still suffering from a prolapse? | ○ | ○ | ○ |
| Do you notice any progress in your pelvic floor muscles? | ○ | ○ | ○ |

## Based on My Self-Analysis:

These are the goals for the following block:

_____

_____

_____

This is how I am going to do that:

_____

_____

_____

_____

# BLOCK 5: WEEKS 13–15

These weeks, the focus is on your lower back to also strengthen your power-house from the rear.

▶ Open your app and join in with the training

**Pre-Workout**
**10 x XL Breath**
**BTY Kegel:** 10 x 5 sec
**Warm-Up:** Foam Rolling, Namaste, Aerobiclike

## WORKOUT

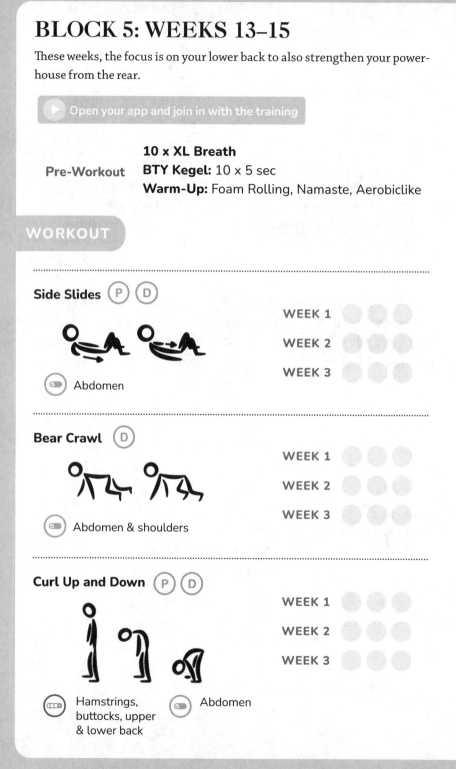

**Side Slides** Ⓟ Ⓓ

WEEK 1
WEEK 2
WEEK 3

Abdomen

**Bear Crawl** Ⓓ

WEEK 1
WEEK 2
WEEK 3

Abdomen & shoulders

**Curl Up and Down** Ⓟ Ⓓ

WEEK 1
WEEK 2
WEEK 3

Hamstrings, buttocks, upper & lower back

Abdomen

## Super Mom (D)

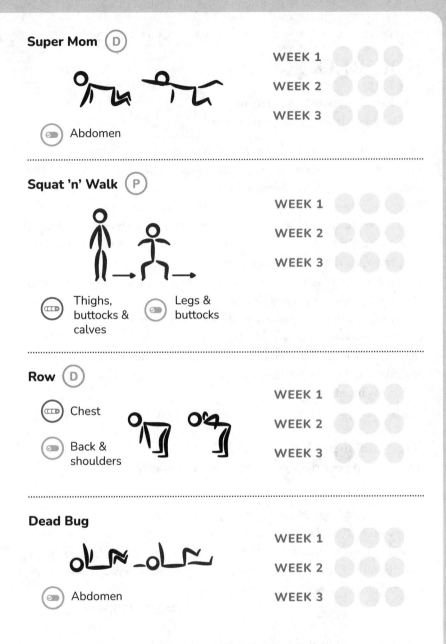

- Abdomen

WEEK 1
WEEK 2
WEEK 3

## Squat 'n' Walk (P)

- Thighs, buttocks & calves
- Legs & buttocks

WEEK 1
WEEK 2
WEEK 3

## Row (D)

- Chest
- Back & shoulders

WEEK 1
WEEK 2
WEEK 3

## Dead Bug

- Abdomen

WEEK 1
WEEK 2
WEEK 3

**Cool Down:** Stretch neck, shoulders, legs

Circle: o = roll loose / o = activate
Add an arrow where you need to pay attention to
your neutral posture

# YOUR XL FUNDAMENTALS FOR BLOCK 5

## XL Fundamental: Nutrition
**Chew, chew, then chew some more**

Digestion starts in your mouth. When you chew, the food mixes with your saliva. It doesn't sound very nice, but it's a valuable process because the enzymes in your spit break down the starches. This makes your food easily digestible. When you chew properly, you release even more saliva, which is good for your teeth. Saliva, in fact, neutralizes the acids and kills bacteria in your mouth. And there's a third benefit: when your mouth is working hard, your brain gets the signal of "being full" much quicker. Therefore, when you chew properly, you automatically eat less. And if that's not enough, a fourth benefit is that chewing is good for brain activity.

Pay extra attention to how you chew during these weeks. Chew a little longer than you normally would. Don't just bite and swallow, but bite, chew, chew, and chew until the food is almost liquid and then swallow it. After a few days you'll notice you automatically chew for longer. It's a simple trick with many benefits!

DONE? YES ⬤ NO ⬤

## XL Fundamental: Rest and Relaxation
**Write down your daily blessings and moments of happiness**

When you write down the nice things in life, you become more aware of your emotions, blessings, and the things you really enjoy. During these weeks, every weekend you should try to write down five things that make you happy, four things you are grateful for, three things that made you laugh, two things you are proud of, and one compliment to yourself because you are a fabulous human being!

DONE? YES ⬤ NO ⬤

## XL Fundamental: Posture and Breathing
**Imitate your baby**

**LARS MAK, musical star and vocal coach:**
Your posture, breathing, and voice are all connected to each other. I am constantly aware of them when I perform. Mimicking your baby is a terrific way

to experience how your voice, posture, and breathing influence each other. Imitate all the new sounds they make—so, all the crazy and funny noises, including screams, cries, and sighs. Your baby doesn't think about what they are doing, so when you do it, you'll feel how naturally your whole body joins in to produce these sounds. And when you look at your baby, you will be able to see how crying or yelling (or, in singing: belting) puts pressure on the abdominal cavity. You see the belly getting rounder, which lets you know the air pressure is increasing.

DONE?   YES ⬤   NO ⬤

## XL Fundamental: Exercise and Training
### More steps than last week

These weeks are marked by getting those steps in. We're not talking about strolling but walking at a brisk pace. See how many steps you walked last week and do more steps this week. Next week, do the same and increase your steps again. In the third week, we crank things up a notch. It's excellent for your health in all manner of ways, from your muscles to your blood circulation to the calm in your head.

DONE?   YES ⬤   NO ⬤

**NOTES:**

_____

_____

_____

_____

_____

_____

_____

# DIARY: BLOCK 5

Time for self-analysis. Fill in after you complete Block 5.

## Nutrition

| *How are you getting on with:* | VERY WELL | GOOD | COULD BE BETTER | BADLY |
|---|---|---|---|---|
| Eating healthy food? | ○ | ○ | ○ | ○ |
| Balancing protein, fat, and carbohydrates? | ○ | ○ | ○ | ○ |
| Drinking 1.5 liters of water daily? | ○ | ○ | ○ | ○ |
| Spreading out eating throughout the day? | ○ | ○ | ○ | ○ |

## Rest and Relaxation

| *How are you getting on with:* | AARGH | GOOD |
|---|---|---|
| Your inner levels of rest? | | |
| The demands you place on yourself? | | |
| Letting others help you? | | |
| Maintaining an overview? | | |
| Getting enough sleep? | | |

## Posture and Breathing

| *Do you pay attention to:* | YES | REGULARLY | NOT ENOUGH | NO |
|---|---|---|---|---|
| Maintaining a good neutral posture all day? | ○ | ○ | ○ | ○ |
| Good posture when lifting your baby? | ○ | ○ | ○ | ○ |
| Good XL Breathing? | ○ | ○ | ○ | ○ |
| Using XL Breath when lifting? | ○ | ○ | ○ | ○ |

## Exercise and Training

| | YES | REGULARLY | NOT ENOUGH | NO |
|---|---|---|---|---|
| Do you notice progress during the training sessions? | ○ | ○ | ○ | ○ |

How many steps do you manage to do a day?

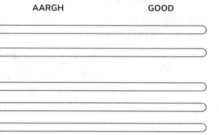

0 steps        Minimum goal: 10,000        15,000

## General Questions

*How are you getting on with:*          AARGH                    GOOD

Your hormones?

The bond with your child?

Your relationship?

Intimate contact?

Social life?

Work?

## Pelvic Floor Muscles and Abdominal Muscle Checkup

*How often do you do the:*          NEVER                    EVERY DAY

BTY Kegel?

XL Breath?

> **Reminder:** Before starting the next block, check yourself for knots in your pelvic floor muscles (see page 143). If you find any, get rid of them first before continuing with your daily BTY Kegel exercises!

|  | YES | A LITTLE | NO |
|---|---|---|---|
| Are you still suffering from a large diastasis? | ○ | ○ | ○ |
| Are you still suffering from a prolapse? | ○ | ○ | ○ |
| Do you notice any progress in your pelvic floor muscles? | ○ | ○ | ○ |

## Based on My Self-Analysis:

These are the goals for the following block:

_____

_____

_____

This is how I am going to do that:

_____

_____

_____

_____

# BLOCK 6: WEEKS 16–18

Many of these exercises are "static hold": you stay in one position and you need to keep it up—and this is all to get your strength back.

▶ Open your app and join in with the training

**Pre-Workout**
**10 x XL Breath**
**BTY Kegel:** 10 x 5 sec
**Warm-Up:** Foam Rolling and PF Lift 1 + 2

## WORKOUT

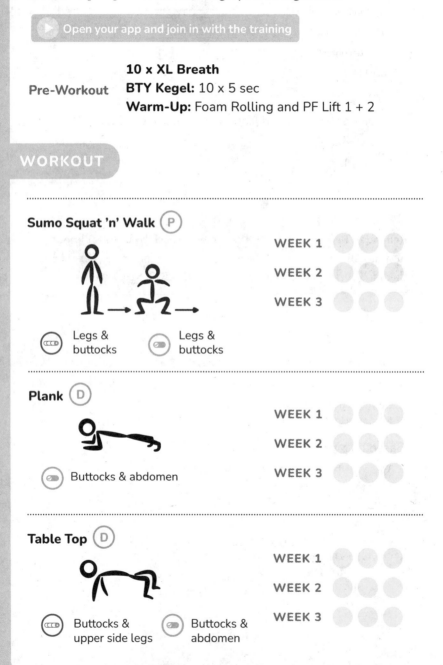

**Sumo Squat 'n' Walk** (P)

Legs & buttocks    Legs & buttocks

WEEK 1
WEEK 2
WEEK 3

**Plank** (D)

Buttocks & abdomen

WEEK 1
WEEK 2
WEEK 3

**Table Top** (D)

Buttocks & upper side legs    Buttocks & abdomen

WEEK 1
WEEK 2
WEEK 3

## Hip Abductor  (D)

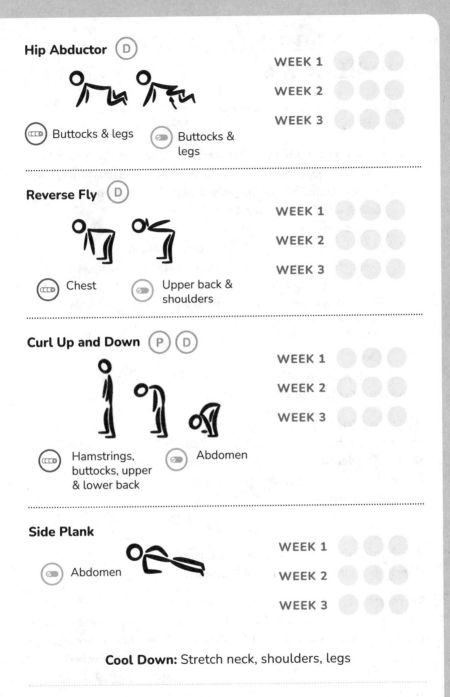

Buttocks & legs

Buttocks & legs

WEEK 1

WEEK 2

WEEK 3

## Reverse Fly  (D)

Chest

Upper back & shoulders

WEEK 1

WEEK 2

WEEK 3

## Curl Up and Down  (P) (D)

Hamstrings, buttocks, upper & lower back

Abdomen

WEEK 1

WEEK 2

WEEK 3

## Side Plank

Abdomen

WEEK 1

WEEK 2

WEEK 3

**Cool Down:** Stretch neck, shoulders, legs

Circle: O = roll loose / O = activate
Add an arrow where you need to pay attention to
your neutral posture

# YOUR XL FUNDAMENTALS FOR BLOCK 6

## XL Fundamental: Nutrition
**Eat mindfully**

You can grab a quick bite in between the errands in your day, but you can also eat consciously and get more out of your meal. Give yourself (and your family!) the chance to eat mindfully during these weeks. You do that by:

1. Eating at the table, all together
2. Taking your time
3. Listening to calming music while cooking and eating
4. Keeping all cell phones and other screens out of reach
5. Consciously chewing your food
6. With every product, asking yourself whether the product is good for your body and mind.

DONE?  YES  ◯  NO  ◯

## XL Fundamental: Rest and Relaxation
**A moment for your looks**

It's so extremely easy to neglect yourself as a mother. The day flies by faster than ever and there's no time to have a decent shower. Allow yourself some time for you during these weeks. Give yourself a hair mask, take an extra-long bath, or pamper your skin with a natural homemade scrub of oil and sugar! You deserve it!

DONE?  YES  ◯  NO  ◯

## XL Fundamental: Posture and Breathing
**Check your shoes: do you walk straight?**

The position of your feet and your powerhouse are connected to each other. If you walk with your feet turned inward or outward, you put disproportionate pressure on your powerhouse. Check the soles of your shoes to see whether you walk properly or not. Is one side worn away more than the other?

DONE?  YES  ◯  NO  ◯

# XL Fundamental: Exercise and Training
## 30-minute vitamin D sunbathing

During these three weeks, try to get outside for an hour every day, preferably by going for a walk. Do it between 11 a.m. and 3 p.m. because the position of the sun will allow your body to make enough vitamin D. The more uncovered your body is, the more vitamin D it can produce (but, of course, be sure to use sunscreen).

DONE?   YES ⬤   NO ⬤

## TIP

Are you not progressing as quickly as you had hoped? Is your prolapse still causing you discomfort and are you unable to gain control of your pelvic floor muscles? If so, see a pelvic floor specialist and get them to see whether the birth caused any damage to the levator ani. It sounds scary, but this muscle sometimes tears partially loose during childbirth. The muscle can't be reattached, but by training the surrounding muscles (the exercises from the BTY program help with that), you can minimize the symptoms. A pelvic floor specialist can tell what you should do in your specific case.

## NOTES:

# DIARY: BLOCK 6

Time for self-analysis. Fill in after you complete Block 6.

## Nutrition

| *How are you getting on with:* | VERY WELL | GOOD | COULD BE BETTER | BADLY |
|---|---|---|---|---|
| Eating healthy food? | ◯ | ◯ | ◯ | ◯ |
| Balancing protein, fat, and carbohydrates? | ◯ | ◯ | ◯ | ◯ |
| Drinking 1.5 liters of water daily? | ◯ | ◯ | ◯ | ◯ |
| Spreading out eating throughout the day? | ◯ | ◯ | ◯ | ◯ |

## Rest and Relaxation

| *How are you getting on with:* | AARGH | GOOD |
|---|---|---|
| Your inner levels of rest? | | |
| The demands you place on yourself? | | |
| Letting others help you? | | |
| Maintaining an overview? | | |
| Getting enough sleep? | | |

## Posture and Breathing

| *Do you pay attention to:* | YES | REGULARLY | NOT ENOUGH | NO |
|---|---|---|---|---|
| Maintaining a good neutral posture all day? | ◯ | ◯ | ◯ | ◯ |
| Good posture when lifting your baby? | ◯ | ◯ | ◯ | ◯ |
| Good XL Breathing? | ◯ | ◯ | ◯ | ◯ |
| Using XL Breath when lifting? | ◯ | ◯ | ◯ | ◯ |

## Exercise and Training

| | YES | REGULARLY | NOT ENOUGH | NO |
|---|---|---|---|---|
| Do you notice progress during the training sessions? | ◯ | ◯ | ◯ | ◯ |

How many steps do you manage to do a day?

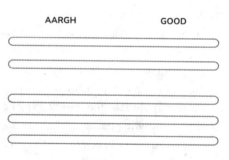

0 steps                    Minimum goal: 10,000                    15,000

## General Questions

How are you getting on with:

|  | AARGH | GOOD |
|---|---|---|
| Your hormones? | | |
| The bond with your child? | | |
| Your relationship? | | |
| Intimate contact? | | |
| Social life? | | |
| Work? | | |

## Pelvic Floor Muscles and Abdominal Muscle Checkup

How often do you do the:

|  | NEVER | EVERY DAY |
|---|---|---|
| BTY Kegel? | | |
| XL Breath? | | |

**Reminder:** Before starting the next block, check yourself for knots in your pelvic floor muscles (see page 143). If you find any, get rid of them first before continuing with your daily BTY Kegel exercises!

|  | YES | A LITTLE | NO |
|---|---|---|---|
| Are you still suffering from a large diastasis? | ○ | ○ | ○ |
| Are you still suffering from a prolapse? | ○ | ○ | ○ |
| Do you notice any progress in your pelvic floor muscles? | ○ | ○ | ○ |

## Based on My Self-Analysis:

These are the goals for the following block:

_____

_____

This is how I am going to do that:

_____

_____

_____

# BLOCK 7: WEEKS 19–21

All your abdominal muscles are going to get a real workout. In this block, you replace the set, basic pelvic floor breathing exercises with a variation with which you learn to use your pelvic floor in positions.

▶ Open your app and join in with the training

**Pre-Workout**

**10 x XL Breath**
**BTY Kegel:** 10 x 5 sec
**Warm-Up:** Foam Rolling, Aerobiclike, and Standing Lizard

## WORKOUT

**Split Squats** (P)

Legs & buttocks

Legs & buttocks

WEEK 1
WEEK 2
WEEK 3

**Downward Dog** (P) (D)

Hamstrings, buttocks, lower back & back muscle

WEEK 1
WEEK 2
WEEK 3

**Sit-Ups** (P) (D)

Lower back

Abdomen

WEEK 1
WEEK 2
WEEK 3

## Hyper Back (D)

Lower back    Lower back

| | WEEK 1 | ○ ○ ○ |
| | WEEK 2 | ○ ○ ○ |
| | WEEK 3 | ○ ○ ○ |

## Dead Bug

Abdomen

| | WEEK 1 | ○ ○ ○ |
| | WEEK 2 | ○ ○ ○ |
| | WEEK 3 | ○ ○ ○ |

## Bear Crawl (D)

Abdomen & shoulders

| | WEEK 1 | ○ ○ ○ |
| | WEEK 2 | ○ ○ ○ |
| | WEEK 3 | ○ ○ ○ |

## Side Slides (P) (D)

Abdomen

| | WEEK 1 | ○ ○ ○ |
| | WEEK 2 | ○ ○ ○ |
| | WEEK 3 | ○ ○ ○ |

**Cool Down:** XL Cool Down

Circle: o = roll loose / o = activate
Add an arrow where you need to pay attention to
your neutral posture

# YOUR XL FUNDAMENTALS
# FOR BLOCK 7

## XL Fundamental: Nutrition
### Herbal tea: perfect for your body after childbirth

Tasty, amazingly good, and easy to prepare . . .

Ginger tea has an anti-inflammatory effect, it's good for your body's acid balance, and it calms your body and mind.

Fresh mint tea is good for your memory and skin, reduces stress, and does wonders for your digestion.

Fresh valerian tea is extremely good for relaxing the mind and body. Take note: you make this tea cold. Yes, that's right. That's the only way to get all the effective substances into the water. Pour 8.5 fluid ounces of cold water over a teaspoon of finely ground valerian root and leave it to stand for 3 to 24 hours. (Again, for some people, consuming valerian regularly can have some unpleasant side effects).

There are numerous other teas that are easy to make, and each one has its own benefits. Because the good substances from the herbs or plants get into the water, the body can easily absorb them. During these weeks, try a different type of tea every couple of days. Amazingly healthy and delicious!

DONE?   YES ⬤   NO ⬤

## XL Fundamental: Rest and Relaxation
### Dry brushing

Start your mornings with dry brushing to give your skin a treat. It exfoliates, stimulates blood circulation, gives you energy, and cleans the pores. Grab a brush with firm hairs and a handle (so that you can also reach your back) and brush your body before showering. Start at your feet and work your way up your body, toward your heart. Move on to your arms and work your way back to your heart. Alternate circular movements with short strokes.

DONE?   YES ⬤   NO ⬤

## XL Fundamental: Posture and Breathing
### Calf time

Your calves are particularly important for your pelvis. Yes, that sounds crazy, but if your calves are shortened, you won't stand properly, meaning you will tilt your pelvis incorrectly. During these weeks, do your calves a favor and stretch them. Stand on your toes on a threshold or raised surface and drop your heels. Do it for as long as it feels comfortable.

Also, a few times a day, stand on your toes and hold it there. This activates the pumps in your calf muscles, which stimulates your body's lymphatic system to discharge fluids.

DONE?  YES ●  NO ●

## XL Fundamental: Exercise and Training
### Sign up for a (team) sport/sports club

It can be tough going, being a mother, and you could feel lonely at times. You will not be the only one. You are home more often, tied to the house more, and your social life is frequently on the back burner. You could consider signing up for a team sport or joining a sports club. It will give you that push to get out for a few hours every week.

DONE?  YES ●  NO ●

NOTES:

---

## EXTRA PELVIC FLOOR EXERCISES!

Now that you have made a good brain–pelvic floor connection and have gotten used to your daily BTY Kegel exercises, you are going to train your pelvic floor in a new way these coming weeks. You are going to tighten and relax the muscles in steps (positions).

1. Breathe in and out three times. With each exhalation, tense the pelvic floor muscles a little more. They will be completely tightened after three exhalations.
2. Now do the same again, but relax them in three steps: completely tightened, half tightened, totally relaxed, and then back again.
3. During these weeks, do this exercise instead of your daily BTY Kegel exercises.

This exercise teaches your pelvic floor that there are different forms of tightening and relaxation, and you will gain even more control over it.

# DIARY: BLOCK 7

Time for self-analysis. Fill in after you complete Block 7.

## Nutrition

| How are you getting on with: | VERY WELL | GOOD | COULD BE BETTER | BADLY |
|---|---|---|---|---|
| Eating healthy food? | ○ | ○ | ○ | ○ |
| Balancing protein, fat, and carbohydrates? | ○ | ○ | ○ | ○ |
| Drinking 1.5 liters of water daily? | ○ | ○ | ○ | ○ |
| Spreading out eating throughout the day? | ○ | ○ | ○ | ○ |

## Rest and Relaxation

| How are you getting on with: | AARGH | GOOD |
|---|---|---|
| Your inner levels of rest? | | |
| The demands you place on yourself? | | |
| Letting others help you? | | |
| Maintaining an overview? | | |
| Getting enough sleep? | | |

## Posture and Breathing

| Do you pay attention to: | YES | REGULARLY | NOT ENOUGH | NO |
|---|---|---|---|---|
| Maintaining a good neutral posture all day? | ○ | ○ | ○ | ○ |
| Good posture when lifting your baby? | ○ | ○ | ○ | ○ |
| Good XL Breathing? | ○ | ○ | ○ | ○ |
| Using XL Breath when lifting? | ○ | ○ | ○ | ○ |

## Exercise and Training

| | YES | REGULARLY | NOT ENOUGH | NO |
|---|---|---|---|---|
| Do you notice progress during the training sessions? | ○ | ○ | ○ | ○ |
| How many steps do you manage to do a day? | | | | |

0 steps

Minimum goal: 10,000

15,000

## General Questions

*How are you getting on with:*                    AARGH                    GOOD

Your hormones?

The bond with your child?

Your relationship?

Intimate contact?

Social life?

Work?

## Pelvic Floor Muscles and Abdominal Muscle Checkup

*How often do you do the:*          NEVER                    EVERY DAY

BTY Kegel?

XL Breath?

**Reminder:** Before starting the next block, check yourself for knots in your pelvic floor muscles (see page 143). If you find any, get rid of them first before continuing with your daily BTY Kegel exercises!

|  | YES | A LITTLE | NO |
|---|---|---|---|
| Are you still suffering from a large diastasis? | ○ | ○ | ○ |
| Are you still suffering from a prolapse? | ○ | ○ | ○ |
| Do you notice any progress in your pelvic floor muscles? | ○ | ○ | ○ |

## Based on My Self-Analysis:

These are the goals for the following block:

_____

_____

This is how I am going to do that:

_____

_____

_____

# BLOCK 8: WEEKS 22–24

It's going to get even tougher for your abdominal muscles, and powerhouse will need to work with the rest of your body.

▶ Open your app and join in with the training

**Pre-Workout**

**10 x XL Breath**
**BTY Kegel:** 10 x 5 sec
**Warm-Up:** Foam Rolling, Dynamic XL Stretch

## WORKOUT

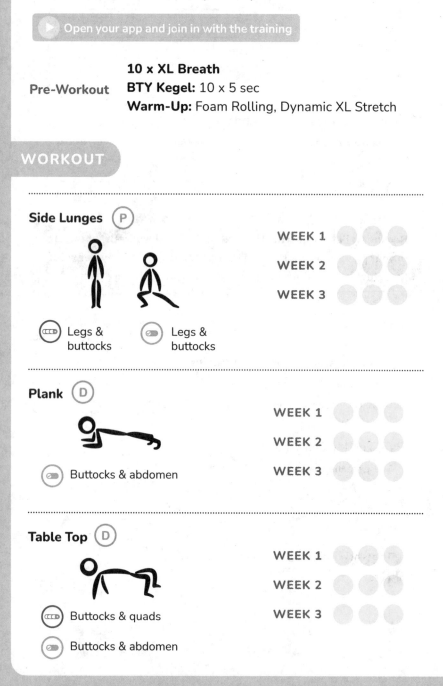

**Side Lunges** (P)

Legs & buttocks

Legs & buttocks

WEEK 1

WEEK 2

WEEK 3

**Plank** (D)

Buttocks & abdomen

WEEK 1

WEEK 2

WEEK 3

**Table Top** (D)

Buttocks & quads

Buttocks & abdomen

WEEK 1

WEEK 2

WEEK 3

**Side Plank**

WEEK 1

WEEK 2

WEEK 3

Abdomen

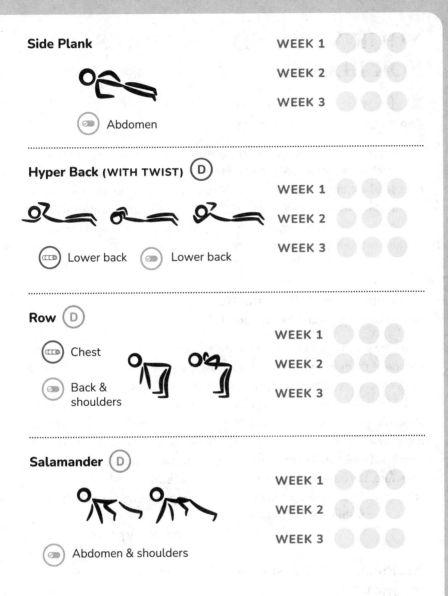

---

**Hyper Back** (WITH TWIST) (D)

WEEK 1

WEEK 2

WEEK 3

Lower back    Lower back

---

**Row** (D)

Chest

Back & shoulders

WEEK 1

WEEK 2

WEEK 3

---

**Salamander** (D)

WEEK 1

WEEK 2

WEEK 3

Abdomen & shoulders

---

**Cool Down:** Body scan

Circle: o = roll loose / o = activate
Add an arrow where you need to pay attention to
your neutral posture

# YOUR XL FUNDAMENTALS FOR BLOCK 8

### XL Fundamental: Nutrition
**Avoid meat a few times a week**

We eat far too much meat and not enough vegetables. Increasing studies are showing that we should incorporate more days without meat in our diet to be kind not only to our body but also our children's body and the planet. During these weeks, try to eat only vegetarian meals three days a week. You will easily ingest your daily 10.5 ounces of vegetables in any case! Make sure you also eat enough grains, beans, nuts, and seeds.

**DONE? YES** ⬤ **NO** ⬤

### XL Fundamental: Rest and Relaxation
**Ten-second time-out for the good things**

There are easy ways to feel happier and more positive, and we are going to try one of them this week. It's an amazingly simple idea. We all enjoy little things every day, but we rarely take the time to allow the positive feelings to really impact our mind. When you take a time-out for 10 seconds to think about the good things, the positive things, the things you enjoy, that positive impression goes from your short- to your long-term memory. This makes you more positive—you'll feel more comfortable in your skin and enjoy life more. Therefore, the next time the sun is shining, take a 10-second time-out and enjoy it. It doesn't matter what makes you happy as long as you hold on to that happy feeling for 10 seconds.

**DONE? YES** ⬤ **NO** ⬤

### XL Fundamental: Posture and Breathing
**Toe gymnastics**

Do you have a bigger shoe size after your pregnancy? Feet can sag during your pregnancy. No amount of training will get your old size back, but it is important that you regularly train the muscles in your feet. Pick something up with your toes. The bigger the object, the easier it is. If you can manage that, try with smaller objects until you are so good at it that you can pile up objects with your feet.

It also helps if you regularly stretch your toes, make a "fist" with your toes, as it were. After tensing them, you should relax them for the same length of time.

DONE?  YES ⬤  NO ⬤

## XL Fundamental: Exercise and Training
### Cold showers

Cold does wonders for your body. During these weeks, rinse yourself off with cold water after your normal hot shower in the mornings. It can give you an instant energy boost. Think about it: a hot shower makes you sluggish and a cold shower has the opposite effect. The number of white blood cells increases when you regularly expose your body to cold, which gives your immune system a boost. Cold water is also really good for your blood circulation, and in turn, your heart and vascular system and your cardiovascular health. See the cold shower as a cardio workout. As if that is not enough reason to brave the cold, it also can help you lose weight.

An exception: You shouldn't rinse yourself with cold water after your workout. After intensive training, you continue sweating for a while and you want the pores in your skin to be open. A cold shower closes them.

DONE?  YES ⬤  NO ⬤

**NOTES:**

_____

_____

_____

_____

## EXTRA PELVIC FLOOR TIP!

Try to tense your vagina without tensing your anus and vice versa. It can be tricky, but practice makes perfect and you will soon get the hang of it.

# DIARY: BLOCK 8

Time for self-analysis. Fill in after you complete Block 8.

## Nutrition

| *How are you getting on with:* | VERY WELL | GOOD | COULD BE BETTER | BADLY |
|---|:---:|:---:|:---:|:---:|
| Eating healthy food? | ○ | ○ | ○ | ○ |
| Balancing protein, fat, and carbohydrates? | ○ | ○ | ○ | ○ |
| Drinking 1.5 liters of water daily? | ○ | ○ | ○ | ○ |
| Spreading out eating throughout the day? | ○ | ○ | ○ | ○ |

## Rest and Relaxation

| *How are you getting on with:* | AARGH | GOOD |
|---|---|---|
| Your inner levels of rest? | | |
| The demands you place on yourself? | | |
| Letting others help you? | | |
| Maintaining an overview? | | |
| Getting enough sleep? | | |

## Posture and Breathing

| *Do you pay attention to:* | YES | REGULARLY | NOT ENOUGH | NO |
|---|:---:|:---:|:---:|:---:|
| Maintaining a good neutral posture all day? | ○ | ○ | ○ | ○ |
| Good posture when lifting your baby? | ○ | ○ | ○ | ○ |
| Good XL Breathing? | ○ | ○ | ○ | ○ |
| Using XL Breath when lifting? | ○ | ○ | ○ | ○ |

## Exercise and Training

| | YES | REGULARLY | NOT ENOUGH | NO |
|---|:---:|:---:|:---:|:---:|
| Do you notice progress during the training sessions? | ○ | ○ | ○ | ○ |
| How many steps do you manage to do a day? | | | | |

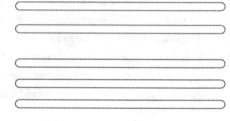

0 steps

Minimum goal: 10,000

15,000

## General Questions

*How are you getting on with:*   AARGH   GOOD

Your hormones?

The bond with your child?

Your relationship?

Intimate contact?

Social life?

Work?

## Pelvic Floor Muscles and Abdominal Muscle Checkup

*How often do you do the:*   NEVER   EVERY DAY

BTY Kegel?

XL Breath?

**Reminder:** Before starting the next block, check yourself for knots in your pelvic floor muscles (see page 143). If you find any, get rid of them first before continuing with your daily BTY Kegel exercises!

|  | YES | A LITTLE | NO |
|---|---|---|---|
| Are you still suffering from a large diastasis? | ○ | ○ | ○ |
| Are you still suffering from a prolapse? | ○ | ○ | ○ |
| Do you notice any progress in your pelvic floor muscles? | ○ | ○ | ○ |

## Based on My Self-Analysis:

These are the goals for the following block:

_____

_____

This is how I am going to do that:

_____

_____

_____

# PHASE 3: YOU

The third and final stage of recovering from the pregnancy and child-birth is kicking off. It is now time to get . . . Back To YOU! From now on, your body and mind can gradually work toward the point you were at before your pregnancy. Your body is stronger, you can start thinking about your figure, and your pelvic floor will have bounced back from the massive attack it endured. You have gotten more used to life with a baby, and even though exciting and surprising things happen every day with a little one around you, and even though your nights are not like they used to be, in one way or another you will find or will have found your routine. Now, you can really get yourself back, mentally and physically.

And precisely now that you are ready for a new phase, motherly guilt could rear its head. When do you put yourself first? How do you balance that with all the attention and love you want to give your baby and family? How can you manage that while combining work, friends, household chores, all the things you need to arrange? And amid all those things, where is the time and space for you?

This is what you can expect in this phase:
- Practical matters: losing weight
- Experts: helpful You tips

FROM SOUL SEARCHING TO TRAINING HARD, YOU WILL BECOME YOU AGAIN, AND EVEN A BETTER AND RICHER VERSION OF . . . "YOU."

## Losing Weight . . . Bye-Bye, Pounds

You've got yourself back on your feet somewhat, and then you see them: those extra pounds you gained during pregnancy and perhaps in the past few months. It's time to lose them, not with a diet but in a completely natural way. If you follow these rules of thumb, you'll notice all those extra pounds quickly disappear, and they won't come back! In these two pages, you can read about the only method and the only diet that will give you a beautiful figure for life. Guaranteed. And that's simply because you adjust your lifestyle. It's much easier than you think and highly effective.

1. Don't diet while breastfeeding and not even in the two months after-ward. Before you can conclude how much weight you've gained, you first have to give your body a chance to get rid of the hormones you produced to breastfeed. At a certain point, you'll notice you suddenly

lose a lot more weight when you are breastfeeding. It's never been proven, but every mother knows, it's like your baby almost sucks out your pounds at a certain point. Perhaps not as many as you would like, but every pound counts, after all. But breastfeeding is not an excuse to eat excessively. Yes, you need to consume a little extra, but that's not a license to eat large portions of food, even if it's healthy food. Keep an eye on what you are eating and your calorie intake.

2. Find out how many calories you should be consuming each day based on your height and daily activity levels. It's generally 2,000 calories per day. Download an app that keeps track of what you eat and shows you whether you are consuming enough (or too much) protein, carbohydrates, and good fat. Keep it up for three weeks and you will get a grip on your eating habits.

3. Have you stopped breastfeeding and think that now is a good time to lose those final pounds? If so, eat a few hundred calories less than you need (e.g., eat 1,700 calories per day if you need 2,000). You will lose a little weight every day, and you can still eat everything. You give your stomach the chance to slowly get used to eating less food, which means you won't feel hungry. When you have lost those excess pounds, you can start eating your required daily calories that you need for your height and ideal weight.

4. Don't skip a training session. You can do the exercises from the "You" phase for the rest of your life. You burn a lot of fat with every training session. Three times a week, no excuses.

5. Eat from a smaller plate. Yes, it sounds crazy, but it's been proven that you eat less. Your eyes see a full plate and your brain is tricked into thinking you've eaten a full plate of food.

6. Have a good breakfast within an hour of getting up. It will prevent your blood sugar level from dropping too low, which will make you hungry.

7. Eat according to the XL Fundamental recommendations. That's eating normal but honest and clean food. The pounds will drop off and you won't put the weight back on if you keep up these eating habits. And that's without even dieting!

8. A moment on the lips, a lifetime on the hips . . . but tackling only your eating habits won't be enough to lose weight. If you really want to lose weight and look toned, you will have to motivate and challenge yourself with the workouts. Try to do as many exercises as possible at the highest level. Grit your teeth, keep your goal in your sights, and go for it!

# "YOU" TIPS FROM THE EXPERTS

## DR. SHEILA DE LIZ, gynecologist, Wiesbaden, Germany

You're back! Totally you and, actually, an even better version of yourself. Or . . . not quite there yet? Check whether you:

- **Are really happy with "You."** Are you happy with the choices you have made concerning your work, personal care, contact with your friends? If not, make some changes right now. As a woman, you need to feel comfortable in your own skin and feel your inner strength. And not only for yourself but also as an example to your child and to benefit any relationship you are in.
- **Have picked up your sex life again.** If not, it's really time to do something about it. Sometimes you just have to have sex a few times to get back into the mood. After one or a few times, it usually gets nicer and you will realize what you've been missing. If after almost a year after childbirth you haven't had sex, well, tonight's the night! *Doctor's orders* ;-).
- **Have kept training and working on your body.** Your body is your temple, and you want to be able to enjoy it for a long time. Your body needs maintenance, just like your looks and mind do. And all this hard work will give you many benefits. Be nice to your body and not only will you feel better and healthier, but you will also have fewer symptoms during menopause and you will still be having sex at age 80. Be good to your body and it will be good to you and any subsequent baby.

## ANN-MARLENE HENNING, sex and relationship therapist, Hamburg, Germany

Science has shown that the greatest sex killer is the length of your relationship. So, be curious and stay curious. Connect and stay connected to each other and to your own body. It may seem that sex is one of those things that should come naturally, but that's not always the case. Sex is determined by the dual control model (see page 47) from John Bancroft and Erick Janssen. And that's why sex doesn't happen as a matter of course for some people and they need to work at it. And remember, use it or lose it also applies to sex. Try to regain your sex life, be true to yourself, and rediscover your relationship. Ignore what anyone else says and listen to your inner sex goddess.

## DRS. MIRANDA GOËRTZ, psychologist, Arnhem, the Netherlands

In the "You" phase, you are actually going to rediscover yourself and your own strength.

- **Setting goals can help.** Ask yourself, what will my life look like in a year? What goals do I want to have achieved by then? Ask yourself these questions before talking with your partner or a good friend. Make sure your wishes are clear. When your goals, your desires are clear, then it will be easier to make better choices that will really help you get Back To You. Look at any blockages or fears you have that are standing in the way of reaching your goals. Take small steps in this process. Focus on the things you can change and not on things you can't control. Focus your time and energy on the things within your circle of influence!
- **Accept that you and your partner may occasionally take the tension out on each other.** Remember, it's due to the circumstances and not an issue with you or your partner.
- **Make sure you have rhythm in your day.** Rhythm carries you through life. Set routines cost less brain power, after all.

# Training in the "You" Phase

You are about to start the final phase of recovery . . . and it's going to be tough going. We are going to do more high-impact exercises that are good for your stamina and muscles, and that will mobilize and stabilize you in one exercise. It's going to get harder from here on in.

### TRAINING TIP

Is your pelvic floor still giving you trouble? If so, repeat the pelvic floor exercises from the "Back" and "To" phases.

## For This Phase, You Will Need:

- Weights (from 2 to 20 pounds, adjustable)
- Foam roll
- Jumping rope
- Elastic band (optional)
- Gym ball (optional)

## Your Daily BTY Kegel Exercises

We are staying at 5 seconds, but . . .

- When you reach 25–27 weeks in the program, we ramp it up a little: for the first time, you will train your pelvic floor while walking.
- In weeks 31–33, it really gets exciting for your pelvic floor: we are going to do exercises while jumping!

Fill in your starting data on page 291 before starting a new phase. It will give you an insight into your progress.

## That Special Week 40

No one can pin an exact date on when you will be fully recovered. One person is back to themselves in nine months; another needs longer. But one thing's for sure: if you can keep up with this workout, then you can do anything! We start this final mega-high-impact week with a special test that checks whether you can jump with a full bladder without leaking any urine. We conclude this week with a very special cooling down. From us, to you. Together, we celebrate than you have come . . . Back To YOU.

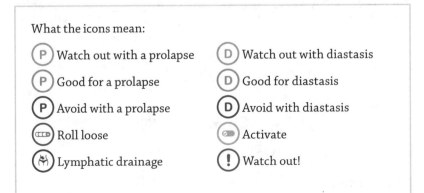

What the icons mean:

- (P) Watch out with a prolapse
- (P) Good for a prolapse
- (P) Avoid with a prolapse
- (⊂⊃) Roll loose
- (🕷) Lymphatic drainage
- (D) Watch out with diastasis
- (D) Good for diastasis
- (D) Avoid with diastasis
- (⊙) Activate
- (!) Watch out!

# BLOCK 9: WEEKS 25–27

Your stability is going to be challenged. You are going to bend forward for the first time again. You are also going to do your pelvic floor exercises while walking.

> ▶ **Open your app and join in with the training:**

**Pre-Workout**

**10 x XL Breath**
**BTY Kegel:** 10 x 5 sec
**Warm-Up:** Foam Rolling, Jumping Jacks (P), and Hip Twisters

## WORKOUT

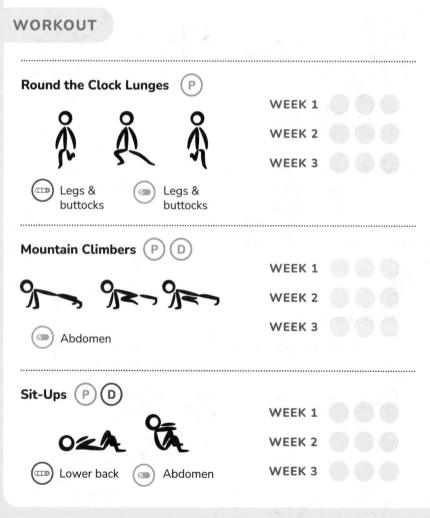

**Round the Clock Lunges** (P)

| | WEEK 1 | ● ● ● |
| | WEEK 2 | ● ● ● |
| | WEEK 3 | ● ● ● |

Legs & buttocks    Legs & buttocks

**Mountain Climbers** (P) (D)

| | WEEK 1 | ● ● ● |
| | WEEK 2 | ● ● ● |
| | WEEK 3 | ● ● ● |

Abdomen

**Sit-Ups** (P) (D)

| | WEEK 1 | ● ● ● |
| | WEEK 2 | ● ● ● |
| | WEEK 3 | ● ● ● |

Lower back    Abdomen

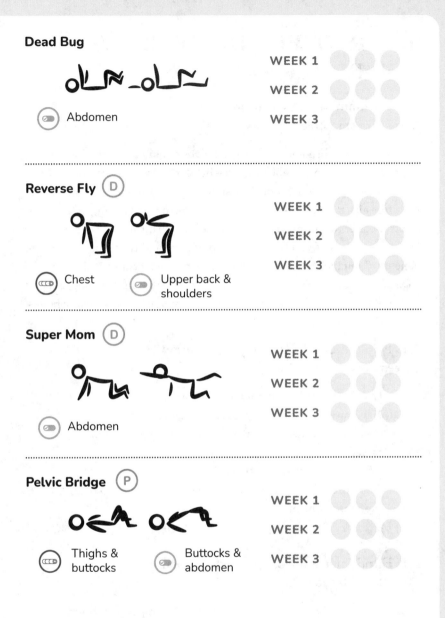

## Dead Bug

Abdomen

WEEK 1

WEEK 2

WEEK 3

## Reverse Fly (D)

Chest

Upper back & shoulders

WEEK 1

WEEK 2

WEEK 3

## Super Mom (D)

Abdomen

WEEK 1

WEEK 2

WEEK 3

## Pelvic Bridge (P)

Thighs & buttocks

Buttocks & abdomen

WEEK 1

WEEK 2

WEEK 3

**Cool Down:** 15-minute walk

Circle: o = roll loose / o = activate

Add an arrow where you need to pay attention to your neutral posture

# YOUR XL FUNDAMENTALS FOR BLOCK 9

## XL Fundamental: Nutrition
**Juices and smoothies**

An easy way to incorporate more vegetables into your daily diet is by drinking them. You can juice vegetables, which will leave you with a juice, or put them in a blender and make a smoothie. A smoothie contains all the vegetable and therefore also the fiber that you partly remove through juicing. In contrast, a juice is easier to gulp down, making it easier to drink more of it. Every juice is filled with lots of vitamins and antioxidants, and those have their own benefits. Combine them, drink what tastes nice, experiment. Alternate the color of your juices, so not always green. Every color has its own unique super-power. When you make a smoothie, add a teaspoon of flaxseed as a bonus. It's good for your bowels!

## XL Fundamental: Rest and Relaxation
**Screen downtime**

1. Give this a go. It is guaranteed to give you more rest!
2. Never use two apps or screens at the same time.
3. Turn off all unnecessary notifications on your cell phone and tablet.
4. Try to limit your screen time.
5. Don't use a screen for at least an hour before going to bed, preferably longer.

DONE?  YES   NO

## XL Fundamental: Posture and Breathing
**The 20/20/20 eye rule**

Your eyes deserve a break, too. Stick to the following rule of thumb: if you have been looking at something close to you for 20 minutes, then you should look at a spot 20 feet away for at least 20 seconds.

DONE?  YES   NO

## XL Fundamental: Exercise and Training
### Always take the stairs

This week, no more elevators, escalators, or moving walkways. Try to take the stairs all the time during these weeks. It increases your heart rate, meaning you will need more oxygen and you'll take deeper breaths. Check that you are using your pelvic floor in combination with your breathing and your movements. Keep breathing, don't push, and do not hold your breath. By doing this type of breathing and muscle exercise in daily life, you train the muscles in such a way that you won't leak urine if you suddenly sneeze.

**DONE?   YES      NO**

**NOTES:**

_____

_____

_____

_____

## EXTRA PELVIC FLOOR EXERCISE!

Now that you have control of your pelvic floor muscles, it's time for another challenge. We are moving from static exercises (standing still or lying still) to dynamic exercises in the form of walking.

1. Stand with your feet firmly on the floor, in a neutral posture.
2. Breathe in and, on your exhalation, tense your pelvic floor muscles.
3. Walk a little without losing the tension.
4. In your diary, note how far you could walk at the start of this block and again at the end of this block.
5. The less often you wear heels and the smoother you walk, the easier this exercise is. The more often you wear heels and the jerkier your movements when you walk, the more difficult this exercise is.

# DIARY: BLOCK 9

Time for self-analysis. Fill in after you complete Block 9.

## Nutrition

| How are you getting on with: | VERY WELL | GOOD | COULD BE BETTER | BADLY |
|---|---|---|---|---|
| Eating healthy food? | ○ | ○ | ○ | ○ |
| Balancing protein, fat, and carbohydrates? | ○ | ○ | ○ | ○ |
| Drinking 1.5 liters of water daily? | ○ | ○ | ○ | ○ |
| Spreading out eating throughout the day? | ○ | ○ | ○ | ○ |

## Rest and Relaxation

| How are you getting on with: | AARGH | GOOD |
|---|---|---|
| Your inner levels of rest? | | |
| The demands you place on yourself? | | |
| Letting others help you? | | |
| Maintaining an overview? | | |
| Getting enough sleep? | | |

## Posture and Breathing

| Do you pay attention to: | YES | REGULARLY | NOT ENOUGH | NO |
|---|---|---|---|---|
| Maintaining a good neutral posture all day? | ○ | ○ | ○ | ○ |
| Good posture when lifting your baby? | ○ | ○ | ○ | ○ |
| Good XL Breathing? | ○ | ○ | ○ | ○ |
| Using XL Breath when lifting? | ○ | ○ | ○ | ○ |

## Exercise and Training

| | YES | REGULARLY | NOT ENOUGH | NO |
|---|---|---|---|---|
| Do you notice progress during the training sessions? | ○ | ○ | ○ | ○ |
| How many steps do you manage to do a day? | | | | |

0 steps

Minimum goal: 10,000

15,000

## General Questions

*How are you getting on with:*

| | AARGH | GOOD |
|---|---|---|
| Your hormones? | | |
| The bond with your child? | | |
| Your relationship? | | |
| Intimate contact? | | |
| Social life? | | |
| Work? | | |

## Pelvic Floor Muscles and Abdominal Muscle Checkup

*How often do you do the:*

| | NEVER | EVERY DAY |
|---|---|---|
| BTY Kegel? | | |
| XL Breath? | | |

**Reminder:** Before starting the next block, check yourself for knots in your pelvic floor muscles (see page 143). If you find any, get rid of them first before continuing with your daily BTY Kegel exercises!

| | YES | A LITTLE | NO |
|---|---|---|---|
| Are you still suffering from a large diastasis? | ○ | ○ | ○ |
| Are you still suffering from a prolapse? | ○ | ○ | ○ |
| Do you notice any progress in your pelvic floor muscles? | ○ | ○ | ○ |

## Based on My Self-Analysis:

These are the goals for the following block:

_____

_____

This is how I am going to do that:

_____

_____

_____

# BLOCK 10: WEEKS 28–30

It's going to get really challenging and tough going—do as many exercises as you can at level 3. During this training block, we will be doing fewer than three powerhouse exercises for the first time, but you will be doing a more difficult variation of your basic pelvic floor exercises.

▶ Open your app and join in with the training

**Pre-Workout**

**10 x XL Breath**
**BTY Kegel:** 10 x 5 sec
**Warm-Up:** Foam Rolling, Jumping Rope (P), and Hip Twisters

## WORKOUT

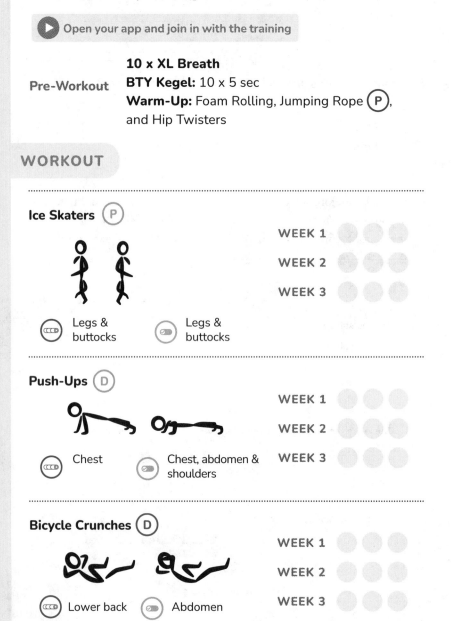

**Ice Skaters** (P)

WEEK 1 ⬤⬤⬤
WEEK 2 ⬤⬤⬤
WEEK 3 ⬤⬤⬤

Legs & buttocks · Legs & buttocks

**Push-Ups** (D)

WEEK 1 ⬤⬤⬤
WEEK 2 ⬤⬤⬤
WEEK 3 ⬤⬤⬤

Chest · Chest, abdomen & shoulders

**Bicycle Crunches** (D)

WEEK 1 ⬤⬤⬤
WEEK 2 ⬤⬤⬤
WEEK 3 ⬤⬤⬤

Lower back · Abdomen

## Triceps Dip (P)

- ⊂⊃ Chest
- ⊂⊃ Shoulders

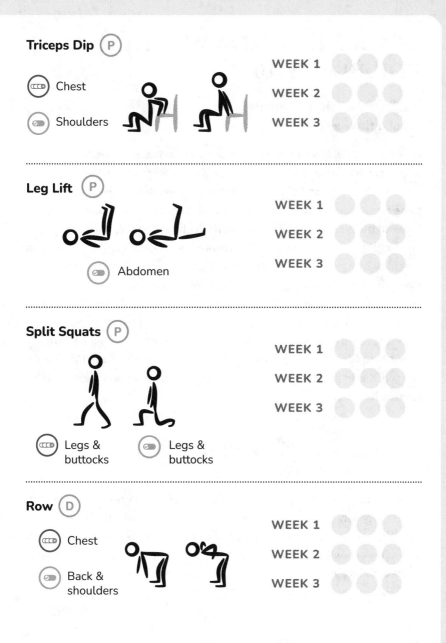

**WEEK 1** ○ ○ ○
**WEEK 2** ○ ○ ○
**WEEK 3** ○ ○ ○

## Leg Lift (P)

- ⊂⊃ Abdomen

**WEEK 1** ○ ○ ○
**WEEK 2** ○ ○ ○
**WEEK 3** ○ ○ ○

## Split Squats (P)

- ⊂⊃ Legs & buttocks
- ⊂⊃ Legs & buttocks

**WEEK 1** ○ ○ ○
**WEEK 2** ○ ○ ○
**WEEK 3** ○ ○ ○

## Row (D)

- ⊂⊃ Chest
- ⊂⊃ Back & shoulders

**WEEK 1** ○ ○ ○
**WEEK 2** ○ ○ ○
**WEEK 3** ○ ○ ○

**Cool Down:** 15-minute walk

Circle: o = roll loose / o = activate
Add an arrow where you need to pay attention to
your neutral posture

# YOUR XL FUNDAMENTALS FOR BLOCK 10

## XL Fundamental: Nutrition
**Ground flaxseed**

Ground flaxseed is a superfood that can do wonders for your bowel movements, and it also contains tons of omega-3 (good for your heart and the blood vessels). The body can't digest whole flaxseed, and it leaves your body in the same form it went in. Ground flaxseed can help ensure the fibers from the flaxseed fill themselves up with fluid in the intestines. Your intestines are encouraged to empty themselves. Or, in other words, you can poop easier and the intestines clean themselves better. This is very beneficial for your pelvic floor, which you can damage if your stools are too hard. It's counterproductive to train your pelvic floor while you have constipation. That is why smooth bowel movements are so important. The seeds have a nutty, slightly bitter taste and are easy to add to salads or a smoothie or sprinkle on a sandwich. About ⅛ to ⅓ cup of ground flaxseed can do wonders for you. (Check with your doctor first, though, if you are nursing or if you are taking any prescription medication.)

**DONE? YES    NO**

## XL Fundamental: Rest and Relaxation
**Time for your social life**

Some moms have it all worked out—a filled schedule and never feeling alone. That is only a small group. As a new mom, it can be extremely difficult to keep up with your social calendar. During these weeks, try to do a nice activity with someone every week. Go to the theater, out to dinner, to a museum, shopping. It doesn't matter what you do as long as you enjoy yourself and spend some time chatting with a friend.

**DONE? YES    NO**

## XL Fundamental: Exercise and Training
**Booty weeks**

These weeks are about getting a nicely rounded butt. Do the training three times a week and apply these life hacks for three weeks. Take a photo before and after, and you will be pleasantly surprised by the results!

1. When taking the stairs, skip one step each time when going upstairs. It will take a bit of getting used to at first, but it's highly effective!
2. With every step you take, tense your butt, particularly when your leg is at its rearmost point.
3. When you are standing still, tense your butt really hard, hold for three seconds, and then relax for three seconds. Do this 10 times in a row.

**DONE?   YES        NO**

**NOTES:**

_____

_____

_____

_____

_____

_____

_____

_____

_____

# DIARY: BLOCK 10

Time for self-analysis. Fill in after you complete Block 10.

## Nutrition

| *How are you getting on with:* | VERY WELL | GOOD | COULD BE BETTER | BADLY |
|---|---|---|---|---|
| Eating healthy food? | ○ | ○ | ○ | ○ |
| Balancing protein, fat, and carbohydrates? | ○ | ○ | ○ | ○ |
| Drinking 1.5 liters of water daily? | ○ | ○ | ○ | ○ |
| Spreading out eating throughout the day? | ○ | ○ | ○ | ○ |

## Rest and Relaxation

| *How are you getting on with:* | AARGH | GOOD |
|---|---|---|
| Your inner levels of rest? | ⟨──────────────────⟩ | |
| The demands you place on yourself? | ⟨──────────────────⟩ | |
| Letting others help you? | ⟨──────────────────⟩ | |
| Maintaining an overview? | ⟨──────────────────⟩ | |
| Getting enough sleep? | ⟨──────────────────⟩ | |

## Posture and Breathing

| *Do you pay attention to:* | YES | REGULARLY | NOT ENOUGH | NO |
|---|---|---|---|---|
| Maintaining a good neutral posture all day? | ○ | ○ | ○ | ○ |
| Good posture when lifting your baby? | ○ | ○ | ○ | ○ |
| Good XL Breathing? | ○ | ○ | ○ | ○ |
| Using XL Breath when lifting? | ○ | ○ | ○ | ○ |

## Exercise and Training

| | YES | REGULARLY | NOT ENOUGH | NO |
|---|---|---|---|---|
| Do you notice progress during the training sessions? | ○ | ○ | ○ | ○ |

How many steps do you manage to do a day?

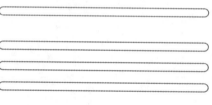

0 steps    Minimum goal: 10,000    15,000

## General Questions

| How are you getting on with: | AARGH | GOOD |
|---|---|---|
| Your hormones? | | |
| The bond with your child? | | |
| Your relationship? | | |
| Intimate contact? | | |
| Social life? | | |
| Work? | | |

## Pelvic Floor Muscles and Abdominal Muscle Checkup

| How often do you do the: | NEVER | EVERY DAY |
|---|---|---|
| BTY Kegel? | | |
| XL Breath? | | |

**Reminder:** Before starting the next block, check yourself for knots in your pelvic floor muscles (see page 143). If you find any, get rid of them first before continuing with your daily BTY Kegel exercises!

| | YES | A LITTLE | NO |
|---|---|---|---|
| Are you still suffering from a large diastasis? | ○ | ○ | ○ |
| Are you still suffering from a prolapse? | ○ | ○ | ○ |
| Do you notice any progress in your pelvic floor muscles? | ○ | ○ | ○ |

## Based on My Self-Analysis:

These are the goals for the following block:

_____

_____

This is how I am going to do that:

_____

_____

_____

# BLOCK 11: WEEKS 31–33

We are going to be doing more and more exercises for the rest of your body, but keep paying attention to your pelvic floor.

▶ Open your app and join in with the training

**Pre-Workout**  **10 x XL Breath**
**BTY Kegel:** 10 x 5 sec
**Warm-Up:** Foam Rolling, Aerobiclike, and Standing Lizard

## WORKOUT

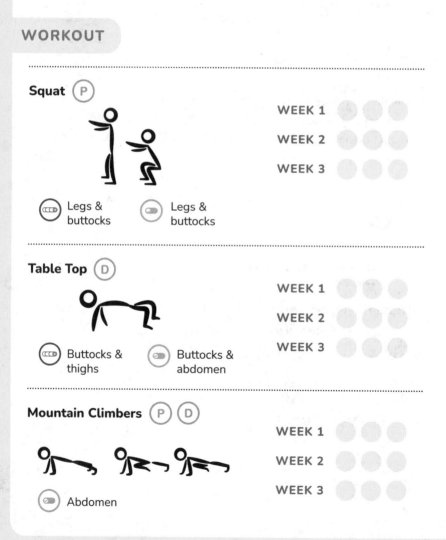

**Squat** (P)

|  | WEEK 1 | ◯ ◯ ◯ |
|---|---|---|
|  | WEEK 2 | ◯ ◯ ◯ |
|  | WEEK 3 | ◯ ◯ ◯ |

Legs & buttocks    Legs & buttocks

**Table Top** (D)

|  | WEEK 1 | ◯ ◯ ◯ |
|---|---|---|
|  | WEEK 2 | ◯ ◯ ◯ |
|  | WEEK 3 | ◯ ◯ ◯ |

Buttocks & thighs    Buttocks & abdomen

**Mountain Climbers** (P) (D)

|  | WEEK 1 | ◯ ◯ ◯ |
|---|---|---|
|  | WEEK 2 | ◯ ◯ ◯ |
|  | WEEK 3 | ◯ ◯ ◯ |

Abdomen

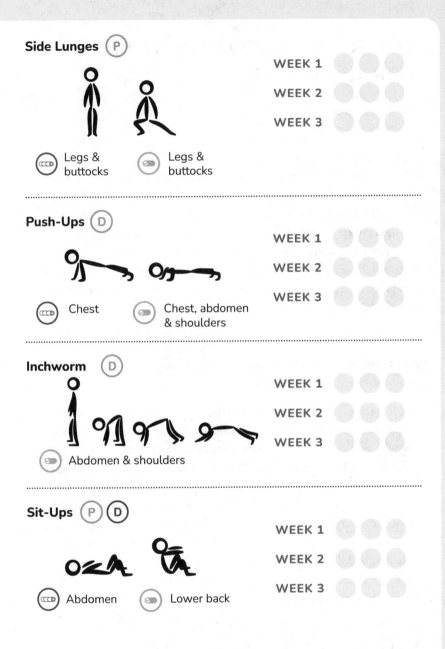

## Side Lunges (P)

Legs & buttocks

Legs & buttocks

WEEK 1

WEEK 2

WEEK 3

## Push-Ups (D)

Chest

Chest, abdomen & shoulders

WEEK 1

WEEK 2

WEEK 3

## Inchworm (D)

Abdomen & shoulders

WEEK 1

WEEK 2

WEEK 3

## Sit-Ups (P) (D)

Abdomen

Lower back

WEEK 1

WEEK 2

WEEK 3

**Cool Down:** XL Cool Down

Circle: o = roll loose / o = activate
Add an arrow where you need to pay attention to
your neutral posture

# YOUR XL FUNDAMENTALS FOR BLOCK 11

## XL Fundamental: Nutrition
**Cut back on bread**

Regardless of the debate of whether bread is good for you or not, we all agree we need a varied diet. In short, two bread-based meals a day is not varied. Try to alternate your breakfast with muesli and yogurt, or with oats. They are excellent for your intestines. Also pay attention to the sugar content of commercially prepared muesli. Most contain a lot of sugar, and that's something you want to avoid. You can make your own muesli in 10 minutes, and if you put it in an airtight container it will keep for two weeks. You can vary your lunch with a soup or salad. Give yourself a great lunch by sprinkling your salad with ground flaxseed and other grains and seeds.

**DONE?  YES    NO**

## XL Fundamental: Rest and Relaxation
**Your earlobes' erogenous zone**

Lots of nerves come together in our earlobe, and many cultures believe they are connected to various organs and body parts. A daily one-minute massage will do wonders for you. The earlobe is sensitive, and touching it relieves stress and almost instantly relaxes you. You can even reduce or get rid of some types of headaches by massaging your earlobe.

First, carefully rub the entire ear to "wake it up." Then pull gently on one ear at three different points. Fold your ear double, first forward and then downward. Make drumming motions with your fingers next to your ear. Now place your middle finger in front of your ear and your index finger behind your ear and make rubbing motions. Grab your earlobe between two fingers and massage it. Instant energy!

**DONE?  YES    NO**

## XL Fundamental: Posture and Breathing
**Work on your stability**

You have come so far already, you are as good as Back To You, but you can always become an even better version of yourself ;-). Training your stability prevents any weak points from causing you health issues later on. And the wonderful thing is, the stability training costs no time at all. For example, stand on one leg while brushing your teeth. Stand on one leg while you are waiting in a line (with the other just off the floor, no one will notice what you are doing).

DONE?   YES ◯   NO ◯

## XL Fundamental: Exercise and Training
### Bring mommy up, bring mommy down

This is going to be tough going, but it's extremely good for your butt and legs. Google the song "Bring Sally Up, Bring Sally Down" and join in with the song. On the word *down* you go into a squat, and on *up* you come up again . . . count down in your head. Do this block five days per week. It's tough but it gives you quick results! If you are still suffering from a prolapse, then this will be too hard for you. Wait until your prolapse has fully recovered. (And if you have knee or other joint problems, you should be doing this to start with.)

DONE?   YES ◯   NO ◯

## EXTRA PELVIC FLOOR EXERCISE!

Once you have good control of your pelvic floor muscles and can do the BTY Kegel exercises standing, sitting, or lying down, and even the walking exercises, it's time for an exercise where you jump.

Stand up, tense your pelvic floor, and start jumping.

Count how many times you can jump without losing the tension. Note it in your diary. Count again at the end of this block. Have you made progress?

NOTES:

_____

_____

_____

_____

_____

# DIARY: BLOCK 11

Time for self-analysis. Fill in after you complete Block 11.

## Nutrition

| How are you getting on with: | VERY WELL | GOOD | COULD BE BETTER | BADLY |
|---|---|---|---|---|
| Eating healthy food? | ○ | ○ | ○ | ○ |
| Balancing protein, fat, and carbohydrates? | ○ | ○ | ○ | ○ |
| Drinking 1.5 liters of water daily? | ○ | ○ | ○ | ○ |
| Spreading out eating throughout the day? | ○ | ○ | ○ | ○ |

## Rest and Relaxation

| How are you getting on with: | AARGH | GOOD |
|---|---|---|
| Your inner levels of rest? | | |
| The demands you place on yourself? | | |
| Letting others help you? | | |
| Maintaining an overview? | | |
| Getting enough sleep? | | |

## Posture and Breathing

| Do you pay attention to: | YES | REGULARLY | NOT ENOUGH | NO |
|---|---|---|---|---|
| Maintaining a good neutral posture all day? | ○ | ○ | ○ | ○ |
| Good posture when lifting your baby? | ○ | ○ | ○ | ○ |
| Good XL Breathing? | ○ | ○ | ○ | ○ |
| Using XL Breath when lifting? | ○ | ○ | ○ | ○ |

## Exercise and Training

| | YES | REGULARLY | NOT ENOUGH | NO |
|---|---|---|---|---|
| Do you notice progress during the training sessions? | ○ | ○ | ○ | ○ |
| How many steps do you manage to do a day? | | | | |

0 steps

Minimum goal: 10,000

15,000

## General Questions

*How are you getting on with:*

| | AARGH | GOOD |
|---|---|---|
| Your hormones? | | |
| The bond with your child? | | |
| Your relationship? | | |
| Intimate contact? | | |
| Social life? | | |
| Work? | | |

## Pelvic Floor Muscles and Abdominal Muscle Checkup

*How often do you do the:*

| | NEVER | EVERY DAY |
|---|---|---|
| BTY Kegel? | | |
| XL Breath? | | |

**Reminder:** Before starting the next block, check yourself for knots in your pelvic floor muscles (see page 143). If you find any, get rid of them first before continuing with your daily BTY Kegel exercises!

| | YES | A LITTLE | NO |
|---|---|---|---|
| Are you still suffering from a large diastasis? | ○ | ○ | ○ |
| Are you still suffering from a prolapse? | ○ | ○ | ○ |
| Do you notice any progress in your pelvic floor muscles? | ○ | ○ | ○ |

## Based on My Self-Analysis:

These are the goals for the following block:

_____

_____

This is how I am going to do that:

_____

_____

_____

# BLOCK 12: WEEKS 34–36

We are going to do more jumping and see how the pelvic floor copes with the force of jumping. We are also going to work on your stamina.

▶ Open your app and join in with the training

**Pre-Workout**
**10 x XL Breath**
**BTY Kegel:** 10 x 5 sec
**Warm-Up:** Foam Rolling, Dynamic XL Stretch

## WORKOUT

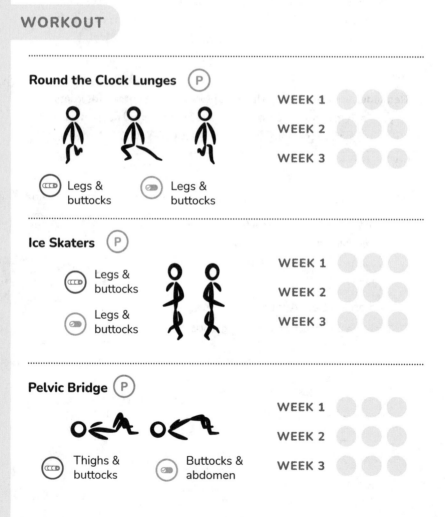

**Round the Clock Lunges** (P)

Legs & buttocks    Legs & buttocks

WEEK 1
WEEK 2
WEEK 3

**Ice Skaters** (P)

Legs & buttocks
Legs & buttocks

WEEK 1
WEEK 2
WEEK 3

**Pelvic Bridge** (P)

Thighs & buttocks    Buttocks & abdomen

WEEK 1
WEEK 2
WEEK 3

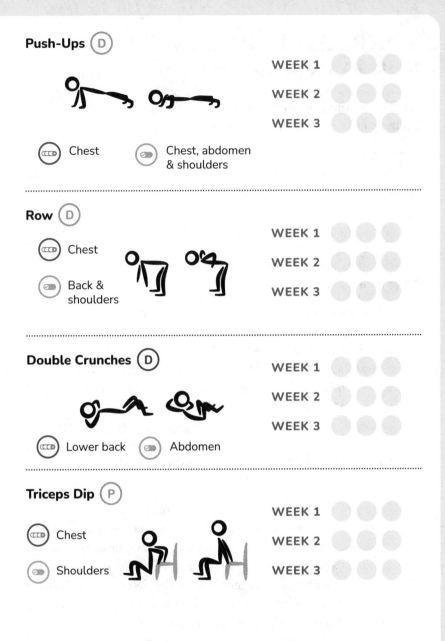

## Push-Ups Ⓓ

WEEK 1
WEEK 2
WEEK 3

Chest

Chest, abdomen & shoulders

## Row Ⓓ

Chest

Back & shoulders

WEEK 1
WEEK 2
WEEK 3

## Double Crunches Ⓓ

WEEK 1
WEEK 2
WEEK 3

Lower back    Abdomen

## Triceps Dip Ⓟ

Chest

Shoulders

WEEK 1
WEEK 2
WEEK 3

**Cool Down:** Body scan

Circle: o = roll loose / o = activate
Add an arrow where you need to pay attention to
your neutral posture

# YOUR XL FUNDAMENTALS FOR BLOCK 12

## XL Fundamental: Nutrition
**Do the check: are you eating the rainbow?**

Every vegetable has its own superpower, and consuming all those superpowers will turn you into a genuine Wonder Woman. A simple trick is to eat the rainbow: red, orange, yellow, green, blue, indigo, violet. Eat all seven colors every week.

DONE?   YES   NO

## XL Fundamental: Rest and Relaxation
**A bedtime story**

Do you have difficulty getting to sleep, perhaps even due to overtiredness? Have a hot bath to help your body relax, meditate for a few minutes, listen to calming music, or read a book. Or even better, do them all. Whatever you choose to do, the aim is to do the least amount of activity, cut out any stimuli, and allow your mind and body to get used to relaxing. You will be helping your body transition from a day rhythm to a night rhythm.

DONE?   YES   NO

## XL Fundamental: Posture and Breathing
**Stretch to the max**

The more your stretch, the more you train your full range of motion. When you stretch, you elongate the muscles, and lengthening is relaxing. You can incorporate stretching in your daily life without it taking up any extra time. Stretch your leg while standing by the coffee machine, waiting for your cup to fill up (it's really good to stretch your inner things because they can pull on the pelvic floor if they are too tight) or stretch your free arm while breastfeeding. In short, find ways to stretch regularly throughout the day.

DONE?   YES   NO

## XL Fundamental: Exercise and Training
### A jump for your lymphatic system

Jump a few times in a row every day. The combination of gravity and your movement gets the fluid in your lymphatic system moving. Do 10 jumps in a row twice a day. Empty your bladder first (reduces the pressure on your pelvic floor muscles) and focus on your breathing. Breathe calmly while jumping so that your pelvic floor doesn't experience any unnecessary pressure or knocks.

**DONE? YES** ◯ **NO** ◯

**NOTES:**

_____

_____

_____

_____

_____

_____

_____

_____

# DIARY: BLOCK 12

Time for self-analysis. Fill in after you complete Block 12.

## Nutrition

| How are you getting on with: | VERY WELL | GOOD | COULD BE BETTER | BADLY |
|---|---|---|---|---|
| Eating healthy food? | ○ | ○ | ○ | ○ |
| Balancing protein, fat, and carbohydrates? | ○ | ○ | ○ | ○ |
| Drinking 1.5 liters of water daily? | ○ | ○ | ○ | ○ |
| Spreading out eating throughout the day? | ○ | ○ | ○ | ○ |

## Rest and Relaxation

| How are you getting on with: | AARGH | GOOD |
|---|---|---|
| Your inner levels of rest? | | |
| The demands you place on yourself? | | |
| Letting others help you? | | |
| Maintaining an overview? | | |
| Getting enough sleep? | | |

## Posture and Breathing

| Do you pay attention to: | YES | REGULARLY | NOT ENOUGH | NO |
|---|---|---|---|---|
| Maintaining a good neutral posture all day? | ○ | ○ | ○ | ○ |
| Good posture when lifting your baby? | ○ | ○ | ○ | ○ |
| Good XL Breathing? | ○ | ○ | ○ | ○ |
| Using XL Breath when lifting? | ○ | ○ | ○ | ○ |

## Exercise and Training

| | YES | REGULARLY | NOT ENOUGH | NO |
|---|---|---|---|---|
| Do you notice progress during the training sessions? | ○ | ○ | ○ | ○ |

How many steps do you manage to do a day?

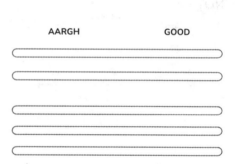

| 0 steps | Minimum goal: 10,000 | 15,000 |
|---|---|---|

## General Questions

*How are you getting on with:*  AARGH  GOOD

Your hormones?

The bond with your child?

Your relationship?

Intimate contact?

Social life?

Work?

## Pelvic Floor Muscles and Abdominal Muscle Checkup

*How often do you do the:*  NEVER  EVERY DAY

BTY Kegel?

XL Breath?

**Reminder:** Before starting the next block, check yourself for knots in your pelvic floor muscles (see page 143). If you find any, get rid of them first before continuing with your daily BTY Kegel exercises!

|  | YES | A LITTLE | NO |
|---|---|---|---|
| Are you still suffering from a large diastasis? | ◯ | ◯ | ◯ |
| Are you still suffering from a prolapse? | ◯ | ◯ | ◯ |
| Do you notice any progress in your pelvic floor muscles? | ◯ | ◯ | ◯ |

## Based on My Self-Analysis:

These are the goals for the following block:

_____

_____

This is how I am going to do that:

_____

_____

_____

# BLOCK 13: WEEKS 37–39

Full body workout and good for your stamina.

▶ **Open your app and join in with the training**

| | |
|---|---|
| **Pre-Workout** | **10 x XL Breath**<br>**BTY Kegel:** 10 x 5 sec<br>**Warm-Up:** Foam Rolling, Jumping Jacks ⓟ, and Hip Twisters |

## WORKOUT

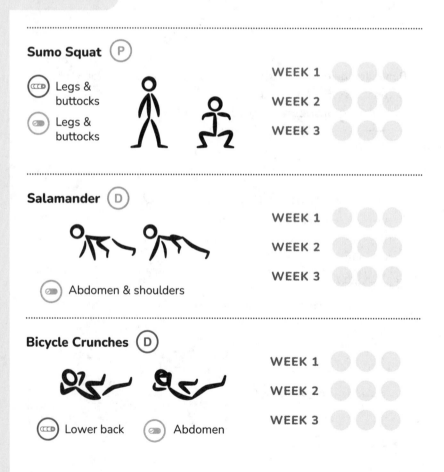

**Sumo Squat** ⓟ

⊂⊃ Legs & buttocks
⊂⊃ Legs & buttocks

WEEK 1 ◯ ◯ ◯
WEEK 2 ◯ ◯ ◯
WEEK 3 ◯ ◯ ◯

**Salamander** ⓓ

⊂⊃ Abdomen & shoulders

WEEK 1 ◯ ◯ ◯
WEEK 2 ◯ ◯ ◯
WEEK 3 ◯ ◯ ◯

**Bicycle Crunches** ⓓ

⊂⊃ Lower back    ⊂⊃ Abdomen

WEEK 1 ◯ ◯ ◯
WEEK 2 ◯ ◯ ◯
WEEK 3 ◯ ◯ ◯

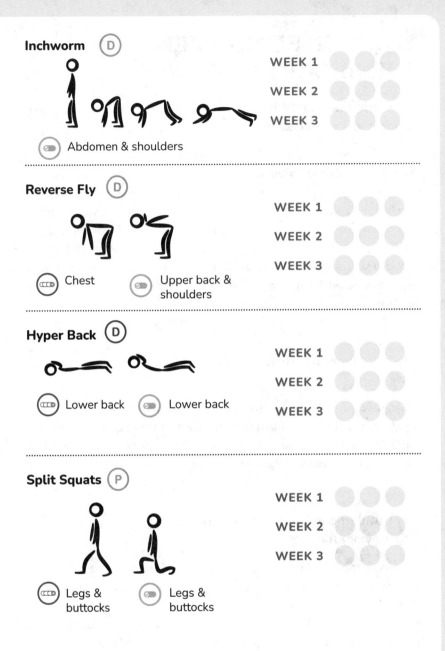

**Inchworm** (D)

WEEK 1
WEEK 2
WEEK 3

Abdomen & shoulders

**Reverse Fly** (D)

WEEK 1
WEEK 2
WEEK 3

Chest

Upper back & shoulders

**Hyper Back** (D)

WEEK 1
WEEK 2
WEEK 3

Lower back

Lower back

**Split Squats** (P)

WEEK 1
WEEK 2
WEEK 3

Legs & buttocks

Legs & buttocks

**Cool Down:** 15-minute walk

Circle: o = roll loose / o = activate
Add an arrow where you need to pay attention to
your neutral posture

# YOUR XL FUNDAMENTALS FOR BLOCK 13

## XL Fundamental: Nutrition
### Lemon water to kick-start your day

During these weeks, start your days with a nice glass of lukewarm water containing the juice of half a lemon. This not only gives you a boost to wake you up, but it also shocks your organs awake, as it were. Furthermore, it hydrates your lymphatic system, contains tons of vitamin C, stimulates your digestive system, and helps if you have heartburn. And speaking of heartburn, if you are suffering from it, dissolve ½ to 1 cup of cider vinegar in water and drink it 30 minutes before your evening meal. It'll help and will do wonders for your digestive system! But all acids, therefore also lemon, corrode tooth enamel. So, rinse your mouth with a sip of water afterward.

DONE?   YES      NO

## XL Fundamental: Rest and Relaxation
### Kissing

Kissing is a great workout for your facial muscles, and it gives you a nice dose of oxytocin. In turn, oxytocin reduces the levels of the stress hormone cortisol. So, during these weeks, give your lips and tongue a workout: it's good for your relationship and your face, and it reduces stress.

DONE?   YES      NO

## XL Fundamental: Posture and Breathing
### Finger gymnastics

This may not be the first body part you think of training, but it is nice to incorporate a bit of finger gymnastics in your routine every so often. Start by hanging your hands beside your body and shaking them until the fingers are nice and loose. Make a fist with your fingers before stretching them completely. Do this 10 times. Now stretch your hand and move each finger individually toward your palm. Next, place your hands in front of you, such as on a table, and lift each finger individually. Final round: place your hands flat against each other and move your palms away from each other while keeping your fingers touching. The tops of your thumbs also stay together. Your fingers are ready to go again!

DONE?   YES ⚪   NO ⚪

## XL Fundamental: Exercise and Training
### An Epsom salts footbath

There is one body part that carries all your pounds around all day and seldom gets a dose of TLC in return. Pamper your feet with an Epsom salts footbath during these weeks. Not only do they deserve it, but an Epsom salts footbath also:

- Relaxes you and reduces stress
- Improves the absorption of nutrients
- Stimulates fat burning (lose weight by putting your feet in a foot bath—not bad, eh?)
- Helps build strong bones and muscles
- Supports the healing of wounds, skin issues, and joint issues

You can buy Epsom salts in a drugstore. (Just don't do this if you have an open cut or burn on your feet.)

DONE?   YES ⚪   NO ⚪

**NOTES:**

_____

_____

_____

_____

_____

_____

_____

_____

_____

# DIARY: BLOCK 13

Time for self-analysis. Fill in after you complete Block 13.

## Nutrition

| *How are you getting on with:* | VERY WELL | GOOD | COULD BE BETTER | BADLY |
|---|---|---|---|---|
| Eating healthy food? | ○ | ○ | ○ | ○ |
| Balancing protein, fat, and carbohydrates? | ○ | ○ | ○ | ○ |
| Drinking 1.5 liters of water daily? | ○ | ○ | ○ | ○ |
| Spreading out eating throughout the day? | ○ | ○ | ○ | ○ |

## Rest and Relaxation

| *How are you getting on with:* | AARGH | GOOD |
|---|---|---|
| Your inner levels of rest? | | |
| The demands you place on yourself? | | |
| Letting others help you? | | |
| Maintaining an overview? | | |
| Getting enough sleep? | | |

## Posture and Breathing

| *Do you pay attention to:* | YES | REGULARLY | NOT ENOUGH | NO |
|---|---|---|---|---|
| Maintaining a good neutral posture all day? | ○ | ○ | ○ | ○ |
| Good posture when lifting your baby? | ○ | ○ | ○ | ○ |
| Good XL Breathing? | ○ | ○ | ○ | ○ |
| Using XL Breath when lifting? | ○ | ○ | ○ | ○ |

## Exercise and Training

| | YES | REGULARLY | NOT ENOUGH | NO |
|---|---|---|---|---|
| Do you notice progress during the training sessions? | ○ | ○ | ○ | ○ |

How many steps do you manage to do a day?

0 steps        Minimum goal: 10,000        15,000

## General Questions

*How are you getting on with:*     **AARGH**          **GOOD**

Your hormones?

The bond with your child?

Your relationship?

Intimate contact?

Social life?

Work?

## Pelvic Floor Muscles and Abdominal Muscle Checkup

*How often do you do the:*     **NEVER**          **EVERY DAY**

BTY Kegel?

XL Breath?

**Reminder:** Before starting the next block, check yourself for knots in your pelvic floor muscles (see page 143). If you find any, get rid of them first before continuing with your daily BTY Kegel exercises!

|  | YES | A LITTLE | NO |
|---|---|---|---|
| Are you still suffering from a large diastasis? | ○ | ○ | ○ |
| Are you still suffering from a prolapse? | ○ | ○ | ○ |
| Do you notice any progress in your pelvic floor muscles? | ○ | ○ | ○ |

## Based on My Self-Analysis:

These are the goals for the following block:

_____

_____

This is how I am going to do that:

_____

_____

_____

# SAVING THE BEST FOR LAST: WEEK 40

The ultimate test of all tests: if you can do this, you can do anything! You are really . . . *Back To You!*

▶ Open your app and join in with the training

**Pre-Workout**
**10 x XL Breath**
**BTY Kegel:** 10 x 5 sec
**Warm-Up:** Foam Rolling, Jumping Rope, and Hip Twisters

## WORKOUT

**Walk-Out Push-Up** (P) (D) (🕷)
(WITH JUMP AT THE END)

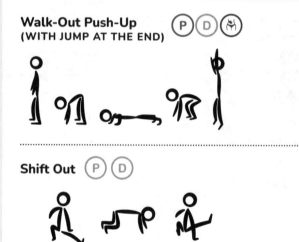

**Shift Out** (P) (D)

**Ice Skaters** (WITH JUMP) (P) (🕷)

(⟪⊡) Legs & buttocks    (⊙⊡) Legs & buttocks

**Salamander** Ⓓ

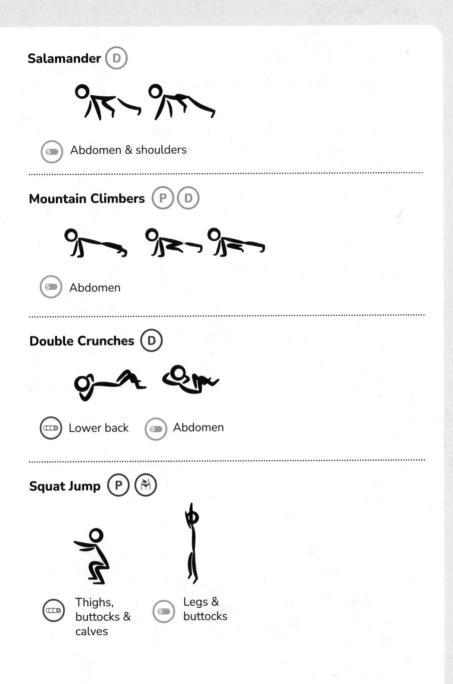

⬭ Abdomen & shoulders

**Mountain Climbers** Ⓟ Ⓓ

⬭ Abdomen

**Double Crunches** Ⓓ

⬭ Lower back ⬭ Abdomen

**Squat Jump** Ⓟ Ⓜ

⬭ Thighs, buttocks & calves ⬭ Legs & buttocks

**Cool Down:** Surprise! Open your BTY app and join in!

# DIARY: WEEK 40

Time for self-analysis. Fill in after you complete week 40.

## Nutrition

| How are you getting on with: | VERY WELL | GOOD | COULD BE BETTER | BADLY |
|---|:---:|:---:|:---:|:---:|
| Eating healthy food? | ○ | ○ | ○ | ○ |
| Balancing protein, fat, and carbohydrates? | ○ | ○ | ○ | ○ |
| Drinking 1.5 liters of water daily? | ○ | ○ | ○ | ○ |
| Spreading out eating throughout the day? | ○ | ○ | ○ | ○ |

## Rest and Relaxation

| How are you getting on with: | AARGH | GOOD |
|---|---|---|
| Your inner levels of rest? | | |
| The demands you place on yourself? | | |
| Letting others help you? | | |
| Maintaining an overview? | | |
| Getting enough sleep? | | |

## Posture and Breathing

| Do you pay attention to: | YES | REGULARLY | NOT ENOUGH | NO |
|---|:---:|:---:|:---:|:---:|
| Maintaining a good neutral posture all day? | ○ | ○ | ○ | ○ |
| Good posture when lifting your baby? | ○ | ○ | ○ | ○ |
| Good XL Breathing? | ○ | ○ | ○ | ○ |
| Using XL Breath when lifting? | ○ | ○ | ○ | ○ |

## Exercise and Training

| | YES | REGULARLY | NOT ENOUGH | NO |
|---|:---:|:---:|:---:|:---:|
| Do you notice progress during the training sessions? | ○ | ○ | ○ | ○ |

How many steps do you manage to do a day?

0 steps

Minimum goal: 10,000

15,000

## General Questions

*How are you getting on with:*  AARGH  GOOD

Your hormones?

The bond with your child?

Your relationship?

Intimate contact?

Social life?

Work?

## Pelvic Floor Muscles and Abdominal Muscle Checkup

*How often do you do the:*  NEVER  EVERY DAY

BTY Kegel?

XL Breath?

|  | YES | A LITTLE | NO |
|---|---|---|---|
| Are you still suffering from a large diastasis? | ◯ | ◯ | ◯ |
| Are you still suffering from a prolapse? | ◯ | ◯ | ◯ |
| Do you notice any progress in your pelvic floor muscles? | ◯ | ◯ | ◯ |

## THE TEST OF ALL TESTS: ARE YOU A PELVIC FLOOR QUEEN?

Drink a good glass of water, make sure you your bladder is full, and jump! Tense your pelvic floor well (of course) and try to avoid any leakage. If you have jumped for a minute and you are still dry, then you have become a genuine pelvic floor queen! If you didn't stay dry, continue doing your pelvic floor muscle exercises. It takes time, but you'll get there in the end.

### Yes, You Did It!

Now, go to page 291 to fill in your final data and see the amazing progress you have made.

# TEST
# YOURSELF

# Test: Stressful Life Events

| | |
|---|---|
| Pregnancy: | ☐ 40 points |
| Gaining a new family member: | ☐ 39 points |
| Major change in financial state: | ☐ 38 points |
| Changing to a different line of work: | ☐ 36 points |
| Major change in the number of arguments with spouse: | ☐ 35 points |
| In-law troubles: | ☐ 29 points |
| Major changes in responsibilities at work: | ☐ 29 points |
| Spouse beginning or ceasing to work outside the home: | ☐ 26 points |
| Revision of personal habits: | ☐ 24 points |
| Major changes in working hours or conditions: | ☐ 20 points |
| Change in residence: | ☐ 20 points |
| Major change in social activities: | ☐ 19 points |
| Foreclosure on a mortgage or loan: | ☐ 17 points |
| Major change in sleeping habits: | ☐ 16 points |
| Major change in eating habits: | ☐ 15 points |

Holmes and Rahe's complete list is much longer, and it describes all major life events. The above is just to give you an idea of the points given to stressful life events that many new parents have to deal with. Look at the life events from the past six months, add the points together, and see how much stress accompanies normal pregnancy and childbirth. If you have over 150 points, you are more at risk of stress-related illnesses. The more points you have, the more vulnerable you are. It's easy to reach that 150 points as a new mother. Every new life event on top can therefore become too much to cope with. Don't forget that, besides being a new mother, you are also a human being. There are no guarantees that you won't be faced with extra stressful situations when you have just had a baby.

The total number of points that you score only gives an indication of the chances of you getting symptoms of stress. Some people function fine, physically and mentally, while scoring 200 points on the stress list. The answer is simple; no two people are the same. One can cope with changes better than the other, and another has a better support network than the other. And we haven't even added hormonal changes into the mix.

# Test: Are Your Pelvic Floor Muscles Strong Enough?

By answering these questions, you will get an idea of the condition of your pelvic floor muscles in relation to potential incontinence.

| | |
|---|---|
| Do you ever leak urine when you sneeze? | ☐ Yes ☐ No |
| Do you ever leak urine when you jump, run, or work out? | ☐ Yes ☐ No |
| Do you ever leak urine in your sleep? | ☐ Yes ☐ No |
| Imagine you really needed to go to the bathroom but had to hold on. Once you go to the bathroom, do you first urinate with a tiny flow? | ☐ Yes ☐ No |
| Is it impossible (sometimes) to urinate with a full flow until the end? | ☐ Yes ☐ No |
| Do you go to the bathroom more than six times a day? | ☐ Yes ☐ No |
| Do you have to get up in the night to urinate? | ☐ Yes ☐ No |
| Do you pass stools more than three times a day? | ☐ Yes ☐ No |
| Do you pass stools only twice a week? | ☐ Yes ☐ No |
| Do you have trouble keeping in wind? | ☐ Yes ☐ No |
| Do you ever leak a small amount of stools? | ☐ Yes ☐ No |
| Do you need to tense to poop? | ☐ Yes ☐ No |
| Do you have piles? | ☐ Yes ☐ No |
| Do you have anal fissures? | ☐ Yes ☐ No |
| Did you have a complete rupture? | ☐ Yes ☐ No |
| Do you have difficulties pooping? | ☐ Yes ☐ No |
| Does your pelvic floor feel heavier at the end of the day? | ☐ Yes ☐ No |
| Do you feel a type of protrusion at the opening of your vagina? | ☐ Yes ☐ No |
| Is your vagina painful? | ☐ Yes ☐ No |
| Do you have back pain? | ☐ Yes ☐ No |
| Do you suffer from overall pelvic pain? | ☐ Yes ☐ No |

### And If You've Had Sex Again

| | |
|---|---|
| Is intercourse painful? | ☐ Yes ☐ No |
| Do you have less or reduced feeling in your vagina? | ☐ Yes ☐ No |
| Are your orgasms less intense than before? | ☐ Yes ☐ No |

**RESULT:** If your pelvic floor muscles are optimally trained, then you would have answered no to all the questions. Yet almost everyone has one or more yeses, especially when you have just given birth. It's no surprise gynecologists across the world are calling out for more attention to this muscle group as part of recovery after childbirth. The biggest issue is that many of the health conditions resulting from a weakened pelvic floor and wrong pressure distribution after childbirth don't surface until years later.

The good news is leaking is not normal after childbirth and you don't have to put up with even a mild form of urine leakage. The BTY pelvic floor exercises will help you stay completely dry while jumping with a full bladder.

# Test: How Big Is Your Diastasis Recti and How Strong Is Your Linea Alba?

Right after childbirth, the linea alba is stretched and even enlarged. The BTY training program will help your vertical abdominal muscles come back together. Regularly check the size of your diastasis and you will be able to see the amazing progress you are making.

## Check the Initial Symptoms: Do You (Still) Have a Very Large Diastasis Recti?

| | |
|---|---|
| You can see or feel an opening or gap between your two vertical abdominal muscles (do the following self-test). | ☐ Yes ☐ No |
| Even long after childbirth, your abdominal muscles still feel weak and blubbery. | ☐ Yes ☐ No |
| Your pelvic floor muscles don't function as they should, and you are unable to train them. | ☐ Yes ☐ No |
| You experience pain or discomfort in parts of your powerhouse, such as your lower back, your pelvis, or your hips. | ☐ Yes ☐ No |
| The region around your midriff feels weak. | ☐ Yes ☐ No |
| You feel pain or discomfort during sex. | ☐ Yes ☐ No |

# Do the Test

1. Lie down on the floor on your back with your legs bent and your feet on the floor. Use a pillow so that your head is raised slightly.
2. Place two fingers in the middle of your belly just above your belly button.
3. With your two fingers, carefully push into your belly while moving your fingers gently back and forth. Lift your head and shoulders off the floor slightly. Stop when your shoulders are just off the floor; you don't have to do a full sit-up. Hold this position for one or two seconds, just enough to do the test but no longer than that. This is not the ideal position for you if you have weakened abdominal muscles or your abdominal muscles are not neatly alongside each other. It can't hurt to test it, but don't do it any longer than necessary.
4. Because you are now using your abdominal muscles, you will feel that they close a little around your fingers.
5. Now, it's important that you pay attention to two things:
   a. Can you still feel a "gap" between your abdominal muscles? If so, how many fingers can you fit in that gap? One or two is normal. And if that is the case, your abdominal muscles are nicely back together and you can train your abdominal muscles. If you can fit three or more fingers in that gap, your abdominal muscles are not back in shape yet and you should adjust the training to help your abdominal muscles come back together. However, there's no need to worry if you measure more than two fingers; it's quite common and can almost always be sorted out through training.
   b. How strong is the linea alba? Can you push down really deeply, or do you feel resistance from the linea alba? You are actually testing the strength and flexibility of the connective tissue. The deeper you can go, the weaker the connective tissue is. It's difficult to express flexibility and firmness in a unit, but compare it to your earlobe or the point of your nose. Ideally, you want your linea alba to feel as firm as the point of your nose.

The flexibility, firmness, and mainly the depth of the linea alba are extremely important because these determine whether your abdominal muscles will function optimally or not.

With this test, you push in your belly. That is why it's important to do it lovingly and gently. It's useless to push hard and carelessly. And it's just as useless to apply hardly any pressure so that it feels like stroking. It is important to find a good balance when exerting pressure. If you are wondering whether you are doing it right, ask a pelvic floor therapist for advice.

**TAKE NOTE:** This test position is not good for you if you have weak abdominal muscles. It's important you do the test, but not 10 times in a row because you would be overexerting your abdominal muscles.

1. Repeat step 5 but now with your fingers about an inch under your belly button.
2. Repeat step 5 but now with your fingers even lower.
3. Note your results in your diary.
4. Adjust your training program depending on the results. Training your vertical abdominal muscles does wonders, but exercising can cause a lot of harm if your body is not ready.

## Various Types of Diastasis

When you did the test, you may have felt a gap of three fingers between the vertical abdominal muscles at a point on your body and a smaller gap at another point. There's no need to start questioning your own test results; this could be completely right. Sometimes the abdominal muscles come back together at one spot, but they still need to close at another.

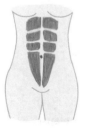 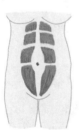 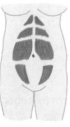 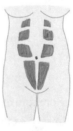 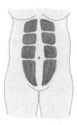

| Normal diastasis | Open diastasis | Open diastasis below the navel | Open diastasis above the navel | Completely open diastasis |

# Test: Are You Suffering with a Prolapse (Sagging)?

| | |
|---|---|
| You feel pressure, pain, or a protruding vagina (bulge) and/or rectum. | ☐ Yes ☐ No |
| It feels as if your vagina and/or rectum is "full" or bloated. | ☐ Yes ☐ No |
| It feels as if your organs are sagging on the outside. | ☐ Yes ☐ No |
| It feels as if you are sitting on a water balloon or ball. | ☐ Yes ☐ No |
| You leak urine (occasionally). | ☐ Yes ☐ No |
| You feel like you need to urinate but nothing comes out. | ☐ Yes ☐ No |
| You occasionally (involuntarily) leak stools. | ☐ Yes ☐ No |
| You have trouble going to the bathroom (constipation). | ☐ Yes ☐ No |
| You feel you need to poop regularly but can't manage. | ☐ Yes ☐ No |
| You have (unexplainable) back issues. | ☐ Yes ☐ No |
| You have (unexplainable) stomachaches. | ☐ Yes ☐ No |
| You can't keep a tampon inside your vagina. | ☐ Yes ☐ No |
| Your vagina makes noises with certain movements because the vagina can't close properly. | ☐ Yes ☐ No |
| You lack feeling in your vagina during sex. | ☐ Yes ☐ No |
| Sex is painful. | ☐ Yes ☐ No |
| You don't feel like penetration is possible anymore because there's "something stuck or blocking" the vagina. | ☐ Yes ☐ No |

If you have one or more of these symptoms, it is advisable to get a physician or pelvic therapist to examine you to see whether you have a mild prolapse. If that is the case, you can do something about it.

# Test: How Do You Breathe?

Do you breathe with your chest, belly, or XL? Using your hands, hold your sides at the height of the rib cage and start of the abdominal cavity. Place your fingers at the front and thumbs behind. Concentrate and inhale deeply. What can you feel? Does your belly move outward? Or your lungs? Or a combination of both? And when you breathe with a combination of lungs and belly, does your belly do most of the work as it should do? See page 106.

# Test: Do You Breathe Optimally?

| | |
|---|---|
| I breathe though my mouth on occasion or frequently. | ☐ Yes ☐ No |
| I regularly yawn or sigh. | ☐ Yes ☐ No |
| I breathe often and quickly. | ☐ Yes ☐ No |
| You can hear a sound when I breathe. | ☐ Yes ☐ No |
| My belly doesn't go up and down when I breathe. | ☐ Yes ☐ No |
| Sometimes I am lightheaded or dizzy. | ☐ Yes ☐ No |

If you have checked one or more of the boxes, then your breathing needs improving.

# Back Mobility: Cat to Cow

Cat to Cow is one of the most valuable exercises for the first weeks when you are working on getting BTY. It is good for the often-shortened back muscles due to you "hanging" in your back during the pregnancy, and it one of the best self-assessments. Watch yourself in the mirror while doing this exercise. Does your lower back move to both sides with your pelvis? Does your upper back move up and down properly? Can you move both parts individually? Does it feel loose?

## TIP

Ask someone to take photos of you from the side, at the same level, while you are doing your Cat and your Cow. Hold the camera in the exact same position. Now compare the positions of your pelvis and your upper back. Did they both move up and down properly?

So many people have pain in their lower or upper back because the pelvic floor cannot move freely. By doing the Cat and Cow in a gentle and focused way, you loosen your pelvis, and this often reduces or clears back issues. You will be able to do other exercises better with a loose pelvis. You will be better at maintaining your neutral posture, and you will get more out of the rest of your training.

If you gave birth a long time ago (or perhaps even recently), this is an ideal exercise to get started with. The process of becoming aware combined with the stabilization and mobilization does wonders for your powerhouse.

When doing Cat to Cow, you are on your hands and knees, meaning gravity pulls on your belly. If you have a severe diastasis and it feels uncomfortable or painful, then you shouldn't do this exercise until you can manage it without pain or discomfort. However, don't give up too easily because this exercise is good for you. Only stop if it really feels extremely uncomfortable or painful.

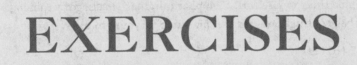

# EXERCISES

Here they are, the exercises that are going to get you into optimal shape. The first exercises are simple but so especially important. They ensure you have the right connection, which will allow you to see real improvements when the exercises become more difficult. These exercises enable your abdominal muscles and pelvic floor muscles to really recover. The more difficult the exercises get, the more "Take note!" notes and variations you will see. Here, you can read why each exercise is good for you, why you do it, what benefits it gives you, what you should pay attention to, which levels there are, and the variations. You don't have to remember it all, of course, because we have filmed each training block so that you can do them at home. Trainer Kathelijne will take you through it all.

## Adductor Ball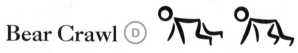

After childbirth (and without recovery, for years after childbirth!), it can be hard to regain control of your transverse (deepest) abdominal muscles. This exercise will be an immense help with that. A nice benefit is that you also activate your inner leg muscles (abductors) while using your powerhouse. Combine this exercise with a lymphatic drainage massage by rubbing over your belly or thighs toward the "big pump" in your groin.

**TAKE NOTE!**
- Pay attention to the natural position of your back. If you can't manage it, then do this exercise in the imprint position.
- Keep your feet and knees far apart.

### Levels:
1. While in a neutral position (body is still), inhale to the count of four, then clamp the ball between your legs while you exhale in 4 seconds.
2. Do the same, but in 6 seconds. Breathe in and out at a pace that isn't necessarily the same as the intensity of your training.
3. And now in 8 seconds, breathe in and out at a pace that isn't necessarily the same as the intensity of your training.

## Bear Crawl

Make sure you have about 16½ feet of space so that you can do a good bear crawl. When doing this exercise, you need to keep all your muscles tense while they work in unison. You must move your weight, and it's not the easiest of positions. It makes sense that it can tire you out, and you can see it is a light cardio exercise. It's excellent for your shoulders and buttocks.

**TAKE NOTE!**
- The starting position for this exercise is on your hands and knees, so you need to take care when doing this exercise if you have a large diastasis. The pressure on the abdominal wall can get too much in this position. Stop if you feel any discomfort or pain.
- Concentrate on your back. Don't let it rise or move downward when the going gets tough.
- Shape is more important than speed.
- Don't make your steps too large.

# Bicycle Crunches Ⓓ

That lovely waistline? You get it with this exercise. You decide how hard you make it for yourself: lying down or with your upper body off the floor. By raising your upper body 45 degrees, you give the top part of your abdominals an even better workout. And if you keep your legs close to the floor, you train the lower part of your abdominals more. But, above all, it's extremely important to rotate properly. The more you do this, the more you use your oblique abdominal muscles.

**TAKE NOTE!**
- Pay special attention to your breathing and do not push. Pushing is extremely bad, especially if you have a prolapse because you put too much pressure on the pelvic floor.
- Try to twist your shoulders as far as possible rather than just tapping your knees with your elbows.
- Do not pull on your neck.
- Make it as hard as possible by holding your stretched leg as low as possible.
- Pay attention to your back: don't hollow it.

## Levels:
1. Almost your entire back stays on the floor, legs fairly high.
2. Legs slightly lower and your upper body slightly higher.
3. Legs just above the floor and only your lower back touches the floor.

# Body Extension

This is an amazing exercise for your posture, and it's great for making space in between your vertebrae again. This originates from Pilates, and it's a great exercise to do at the start of your recovery and throughout life every so often.

**TAKE NOTE!**
Slowly does it . . . the slower you do it, the better your vertebrae can stretch. Make yourself as tall as you can.

# Brain–Pelvic Floor Connection (lying down)

Lie down on the floor in a neutral position. You could place a pillow under your head and under your pelvis for support if you need it. Feel the position of your tailbone.

Now, tilt your pelvis without moving the rest of your torso or your legs. Tilt it upward and move your pelvis slowly toward the floor. Your tailbone will move down and then up. Do it slowly and concentrate on your pelvic floor. Feel what it does when you tilt it and when you breathe. Make the brain–pelvic floor connection.

You could also combine this exercise with lymphatic drainage by rubbing, with your hands, toward your pelvic floor on your exhalation.

# Brain–Pelvic Floor Connection (on hands and knees)

This is a good way to prepare your pelvis for a good Cat to Cow exercise. You can do this exercise if you have a large diastasis, but do it carefully and move to your hands and knees slowly. Don't force anything and listen to your body.

# Cat to Cow Ⓓ

This is the exercise to get your back moving and make a good connection with your powerhouse. This was originally a yoga exercise and is one of the most traditional exercises around. This variant has been adjusted for BTY to obtain the optimal pressure on your powerhouse. If you have a severe diastasis, be careful and stop if it feels uncomfortable or painful. Because you are on your hands and knees, gravity pulls on the abdominal cavity and, in turn, that pushes on the vertical abdominal muscles and the overstretched linea alba. You want to avoid that excessive pressure right now and give your diastasis a chance to shrink.

**TAKE NOTE!**

- Start in a neutral position and return to it in between the Cat and Cow.
- Both your pelvis as well as your upper back should move both ways.

## Levels:

1. Inhale while in a neutral position. Breathe out when moving to the Cat or Cow position.
2. Go deeper and higher than you did at level 1 and hold on to the farthest position for a moment.
3. Inhale while in a neutral position; move from Cat to Cow and back while exhaling.

**SELF-TEST:** See page 265.

# Curl Up and Down Ⓟ Ⓓ

Loosen up those vertebrae. This is a great exercise for your back muscles, and it strengthens the whole lot right away. This exercise prepares your back for the back muscle exercises later in the program that are tough going.

**TAKE NOTE!**

Keep exhaling properly and, if needed, stay still when inhaling and only move on an exhalation.

### Level: Curl Up and Down +

This exercise is actually a self-test in itself. If you notice that you can't curl up and down with a specific part of your back, then you can try to loosen that part with a foam roll (see page 131).

# Dead Bug

This is a genuine all-in-one powerhouse workout, and we bet you are going to feel that. The challenge is in opening up your body completely while maintaining a good posture. This exercise can be really good for you, even if you have a prolapse, because it doesn't put any downward pressure on the pelvic floor. As your arms and legs slowly move downward, they go against gravity, which puts a lot of pressure on your muscles. Keep them tense!

**TAKE NOTE!**

Concentrate on your back. Make sure it doesn't rise when the going gets tough.

## Levels:

1. Arms stretched forward.
2. Stretch your leg when it is low, without touching the floor.
3. Stretched arms and legs.

**SELF-TEST & ACTIVATION:** Dead Bug is tough going for your abdominal muscles, so it could help to activate them first. It will enable you to get more out of your body (see page 131).

# Downward Dog (P) (D)

A yoga classic and an excellent way to stretch your whole body, elongate your muscles, and improve your posture, too. Pull your belly button in and keep trying to point your seat muscles even farther toward the celling. This is the first inverse (upside-down) exercise you do.

**TAKE NOTE!**

- The principle of this exercise is that gravity pulls on the belly. Beware if you have a severe diastasis, and stop if you feel discomfort or pain.
- Don't overstretch your elbows or knees.
- Keep your head in a neutral position between your arms.

See whether the exercise is better, smoother, or easier to do when you first foam roll your upper back. See page 131.

# Double Crunches Ⓓ

This is a two-in-one: you do the normal crunch and leg lift in one exercise. It's effective and saves time. Your abdominals and legs move in and out, and you keep your back in a nice neutral position. It's challenging and great for your lower and upper abdominal muscles. The closer to the floor you are, the harder it is. Let gravity be your enemy. And remember: the slower and more controlled your movements are, the better.

**TAKE NOTE!**
Pay particular attention to your breathing and do not push. Pushing is extremely bad, especially if you have a prolapse because it puts a lot of pressure on the pelvic floor.

You lie on the middle part of your back; when you come up, it is the only part touching the floor, no more and no less!

- Butt just off the floor.
- Do not hollow your back.

## Levels:
1. Arms stretched forward; legs bent.
2. Arms behind your head; don't bend your legs as far.
3. Now with stretched legs.

# Heel Drop Ⓜ Ⓟ

This exercise has the same benefits as the Heel Slide, but this time you move your leg slightly differently in relation to your hip, which means you train a different freedom of movement. Not only that, but it also helps you maintain the pelvic floor muscle coordination when you start using your leg muscles during the exercises. Place your hand on your belly to check you are not secretly "pushing." That pushing puts extra pressure on your pelvic floor muscles, which can be harmful, especially if you have a prolapse. Do you notice yourself pushing? Is your hand being pushed upward during the exercise? If so, then do the exercise at a lower level.

Pay attention to the natural position of your back. If you can't manage it, then use the imprint position.

## Levels:

1. One leg on the ground, one leg goes up and down.
2. One leg in the air, one leg goes up and down. Therefore, you have no support.
3. Two legs up and down simultaneously.

## Variations:

- Press-Heel-Drop-Press: gently push against the bent leg that is not moving toward the floor. This is extremely good for your transverse abdominal muscles.
- When you are more advanced, stretch your leg farther each time. The farther you stretch, the harder it is.

# Heel Slide

This exercise helps stabilize your pelvis because you move your legs, but your pelvis stays completely still. It is a reasonably easy but highly effective exercise. You can increase the difficulty until it's so hard that it almost becomes a leg lift. Concentration is the key to coming to grips with this exercise.

**TAKE NOTE!**

Pay attention to the natural position of your back. If you can't manage, then use the imprint position.

## Levels:

1. Slide your heel over the floor.
2. Slide your heel just above the floor.
3. Now, slide both legs over the floor at the same time, but barely touch the floor.

# Hip Abductor

We all want a lovely butt, and this is a great exercise to work on that. It also helps you get a lot of movement from your hip while having to keep it stable. That can be very tricky after pregnancy because the inside of your legs is often slightly shortened.

**TAKE NOTE!**
- Do not twist your back.
- Don't slouch your back.

## Levels:
1. Move your leg back and forth in a controlled manner.
2. When at the top, hold your leg in position briefly.
3. When at the top, hold your leg in position briefly, stretch it, pull it back, and lower it again.

**SELF-TEST & ACTIVATION:** If you notice that you can't get your leg to move far enough, it can help to activate the muscles first. Try it and see whether you can get farther after activating them. This is how you activate your butt (see page 131).

# Hyper Back (with twist) Ⓓ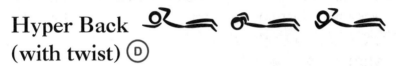

This is an extremely simple exercise. You can do this anytime, and it's good for strengthening your lower back. Do these exercises very slowly to gain the full effect.

## Variation:
You can add a rotation or lift your legs at the same time. You should not do this exercise with a large diastasis because it really stretches your abdominal muscles.

# Ice Skaters Ⓟ

A challenging exercise for your overall fitness and good for ankle and knee stability. And then there's the toning effect. It's a great exercise to get that desired, wonderfully rounded butt. And with this exercise, too, when you can't do any more, do a few more.

**TAKE NOTE!**
- Keep your hips in one line and don't twist too far.
- Do not look at your feet but keep your head in line with your back.

**Levels:**

1. In the farthest position with feet on the floor.
2. With your feet off the floor.
3. So that you feel you are suspended for a moment.

**SELF-TEST & ACTIVATION:** If you are unable to drop down deeply, then see whether loosening your hip (see page 131) and activating your butt muscles (see page 131) will make a difference. After that, does it pull at another spot? If so, loosen that too.

# Inchworm Ⓓ

This combination of moving your body forward and upward is not only great to stretch your body, but it's also a good workout for your abdominals, shoulders, and arms. The farther forward you go, the more you challenge your body. So, go for it!

**TAKE NOTE!**

- Do not do this exercise if you have a large diastasis. After all, you really stretch your abdominal muscles when you move forward, and that is not good with a large diastasis.
- Keep your back neutral.
- Walk forward as far as you can; those final inches are the only ones that really count.
- Keep your legs stretched the entire time.

# Leg Lift ⒫

A basic exercise for your transverse, deepest abdominal muscles, and the bottom of your abdominal muscles. If you have a hollow back, this exercise is extremely good for you because this exercise trains the muscles, making it easier to tilt your pelvis.

**TAKE NOTE!**

- It's a tough exercise, so don't forget to keep breathing. If you stop, you will start pushing, and that is really bad for your pelvic floor, especially if you have a prolapse.
- Avoid a hollow back! If this exercise is too hard for you from a neutral position, then start from the imprint position.

## Levels:

1. With one leg downward.
2. Alternate the two legs.
3. With two legs downward at the same time (only if your abdominal muscles are well trained!).

**SELF-TEST & ACTIVATION:** See whether you can do this exercise better when you activate your muscles first. If so, activate them each time before doing Leg Lifts. If it doesn't make a difference, then just get on with the Leg Lifts without activating your muscles.

# Mountain Climbers Ⓟ Ⓓ

Cardio as cardio is intended—tougher than tough and thereby a helpful addition to your strength training. This is excellent for your abdominal muscles and your whole body because everything needs to be nice and activated. When you think you can't go on, do a few more!

**TAKE NOTE!**

- No matter how tough it gets, keep breathing and don't stop and switch to pushing. You may be tempted when you get tired, but pushing will only make things worse for your body, especially if you have a prolapse.
- Keep your butt low.
- Don't overstretch your elbows.

## Levels:

1. Without a moment of suspension.
2. So fast that you are suspended for a moment.
3. Add rotation.

# Namaste

This is a wonderful exercise to get your chest muscles and powerhouse working together.

**TAKE NOTE!**
Your shoulders should be kept low, and you only use force when exhaling.

## Variation:
Try to clamp a small, soft ball between your hands.

# Pelvic Bridge Ⓟ O🡔🡔 O🡔🡔

When you sit down a lot, the muscles at the front of your hips shorten. The Pelvic Bridge gives you two miracles in one: it lengthens these muscles and at the same time strengthens the opposite muscles, the butt muscles. This gives you a wonderfully rounded butt.

### TAKE NOTE!
- Use the strength from your butt and not from your lower back.
- Only move on to the next level when you can make a completely straight Pelvic Bridge, and not before! You could always film yourself and watch it to check. Most people think they are better at it than they actually are and overestimate themselves.

## Level: Pelvic Bridge +
1. Classic Pelvic Bridge: go as high as you can.
2. At the top, stretch one leg and tuck it back in again.
3. Keep one leg stretched.

## Variation:
Put a weight on your hip.

**SELF-TEST & ACTIVATION:** Try to activate your butt (see page 131) or even loosen it by foam rolling (see page 131) and see whether it's easier to do the Pelvic Bridge afterward. If it is, activate the muscle each time before doing this exercise.

# PF Lift 1 Ⓟ Ⓜ O🡔

This can be a great way to relieve your pelvic floor muscles and ideal for anyone suffering from a prolapse, whether big or small. Not only that, but this exercise also stimulates your lymphatic drainage.

Lie on the floor with your lower legs resting on a stool or chair. Place a pillow under your pelvic floor so that it tilts slightly upward. Close your eyes and feel how your breathing affects your pelvic floor. Do this for 2 minutes. Women with a prolapse will feel instant relief.

# PF Lift 2 Ⓟ Ⓓ

This is a variation of the PF Lift 1 and a good way to relieve your pelvic floor muscles. It's excellent for anyone with a prolapse, and it stimulates lymphatic drainage, too.

Sit on your knees and slowly bend forward. Place your arms around your head so that you lean on your arms. Lift your butt until your legs are at a 90-degree angle. Feel the pressure disappearing from your pelvic floor. Be aware of your breathing in relation to your pelvic floor. Do this for 2 minutes.

## TAKE NOTE!

Since you are on your knees, gravity will pull on your belly. That's fine, but do be careful if you have a large diastasis that is causing you issues. The combination of gravity and being on your knees puts additional pressure on your abdominal cavity and the vertical abdominal muscles, and you could feel that. If you have a large diastasis, your body will tell you whether this exercise is suitable for you and feels okay. This exercise is extremely good for you, but you shouldn't feel any pain or discomfort. If that is the case, skip this exercise.

# Plank Ⓓ

We all know this as the king of exercises for the abdominal muscles, but did you know that this exercise does far more than only tighten your vertical and transverse abdominal muscles? You train your shoulders and back muscles at the same time, and you also work on your posture. Keep your head in a straight line with your body and don't point it upward.

## TAKE NOTE!

- Be careful doing the plank if you have a large diastasis. If you feel pain or discomfort, stop immediately.
- Maintain the plank; don't hang in your back, keep your pelvis neutral.
- Head in line with your spine: not higher!

## Levels:

1. On your knees.
2. Full plank.
3. Elbows on the gym ball.

## Variation:

With stretched arms, lift one leg up, write numbers while planking on the gym ball . . . there are endless variations of the plank.

**SELF-TEST & ACTIVATION:** Try it, and if it works better or for longer after activating your abdominal muscles, then do it each time before you do the Plank (see page 131).

# Wall Pull-Down ⒟

You often pull up your shoulders in periods of stress and add to that the forward-facing-arms position you often adopt. This exercise will work on the opposite muscles, the back muscles, which will allow your shoulders to move back and down and give you a nice open posture. That posture creates a beneficial distribution of pressure in your powerhouse. Doing this exercise against a wall will prevent you from hanging too far backward, which can cause problems, especially at the beginning and if you have a large diastasis.

**TAKE NOTE!**
- Keep your lower arm and hand parallel to your body and not tilted.
- Keep your shoulders back and toward each other, even when it gets tough.

## Levels:

1. Without equipment.
2. With a sweater or towel.
3. With a heavy elastic.

# Push-Ups ⒟

Okay, we know this is not usually a favorite among women, but even though women's chest muscles are often shortened, it is still good to train them. It is important that you do the full Push-Up: so, from bent arms all the way to straight arms. It's up to you whether you do the Push-Ups against a wall or flat on the ground, as long as you bend to the full and stretch completely.

**TAKE NOTE!**
- Keep your head in line with your back.
- Hold your body like a plank: don't raise or lower your butt.
- Don't pull up your shoulders or tilt forward.

## Levels:

1. At hip height, for example a table or countertop.
2. On your knees on the floor.
3. On your toes.

## Variation:

Narrow Push-Ups for the triceps, steps to the side with your hands, diamond shape . . . there are endless variations!

**SELF-TEST & ACTIVATION:** A Push-Up can become unnecessarily difficult if your chest muscles are short. You can often tell because your shoulders will keep moving forward. Try to see whether it helps to roll the muscle loose first.

# Reverse Fly (sitting or standing) Ⓓ

Let's be honest, your body is very much forward focused when you are a mother. Your arms face forward around your baby, and you hold the same posture at your keyboard after your maternity leave. It's time to open it all up with this Reverse Fly. Get those shoulders back and chest open. Stretch those muscles, which have shortened through the cramped posture, by giving the opposite muscle a good strength training. It will improve your posture. During the first weeks, you do this exercise while sitting upright in a chair, without gravity and from a nice neutral position. Gravity exerts too much pressure on your powerhouse and can worsen a diastasis. And besides that, your skin is probably loose and wobbly, meaning leaning forward won't feel very nice. Don't worry, that loose, hanging feeling will go away eventually.

**TAKE NOTE!**

- Keep your upper back and head in a neutral position and do not raise your chin.
- Keep your rib cage still: don't allow it to rise.
- Keep your shoulders low.
- Make sure you go to the furthest point.

## Levels: Reverse Fly +

1. Stand straight.
2. Stand at a 90-degree angle.
3. With a weight or two small bottles of water (Reverse Fly +)

**BEGINNERS REVERSE FLY:** Do the Reverse Fly sitting down during the first weeks of your recovery.

# Round the Clock Lunges (P)

Forward, back, from left to right . . . you go in all directions with those lunges! Feel your legs get heavy and your butt burn. Keep it up for that lovely round and shapely butt. It's a challenge because you must keep changing your balance.

**TAKE NOTE!**

- Keep your head in a neutral position and don't look at your toes.
- Keep your back in a neutral position and don't hollow it.
- Straight lunge: with a bent leg, your knee, foot, and hip are in one line.
- Straight lunge: the bent knee points to your toes, not outward.
- Straight lunge: point your feet forward; keep them next to each other and parallel.
- Side lunges: your knees point toward your toes, not inward.
- Side lunges: your feet point forward and are parallel.
- Side lunges: one knee is under the hip and the other above the ankle.
- Side lunges: rear knee drops to the floor . . . don't stop before you get there.

## Levels: Round the Clock Lunges +

1. Normal.
2. With weights.

**SELF-TEST & ACTIVATION:** See Split Squats (Lunges; page 285) and Side Lunges (page 283).

# Row (D)

This exercise gives you a strong, open appearance, which is the first step to a powerful and open demeanor. Really focus on this part and make the largest possible movement. Feel proud because that's what you look like now. As a bonus, it also gives you a strong lower back. This exercise could soon become too easy for you, but you can keep it challenging by adding a weight. It's good for your posture and whole back.

**TAKE NOTE!**

- If you have a large diastasis, be careful because gravity can pull on you. If you feel pain, stop immediately!

- Elbows as far back as possible.
- Pull your shoulders straight back, not upward, and don't tilt them.
- Keep your wrists straight.
- Stay forward, almost parallel to the floor.
- Keep your head in a neutral position and keep looking at the floor.

## Levels:
1. Standard Row.
2. Row +: with weights or bottles of water.

# Salamander Ⓓ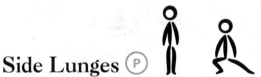

This is a complicated exercise, so there is a chance you may not get it right the first time. Don't give up, though, because this challenging exercise will get you sweating, is good for cardio, and provides controlled and rotating strength from your shoulders, back, and pelvis, and therefore trains your whole body. See it as one of the ultimate all-in-one exercises: a lot in a little time.

**TAKE NOTE!**
- Concentrate on your back. Don't allow it to rise or move downward when the going gets tough.
- Don't make your steps too big: your knee shouldn't pass your hip.

# Side Lunges Ⓟ

The Side Lunges are a great variation on those good old Lunges: a stretching and training exercise in one. You stretch the inside of your leg; the outer leg becomes heavy . . . and can you feel your butt burning yet?

**TAKE NOTE!**
- Keep your head in a neutral position and don't look at your toes.
- Keep your back in a neutral position and don't hollow it.
- When your leg is bent, your knee, foot, and hip are in one line.
- The knee you bend points to your toes, not outward.
- Point your feet forward; keep them next to each other and parallel.

**SELF-TEST & ACTIVATION:** When you step out of the lunge, can you feel you groin pulling? If so, your muscles could probably do with some help to relax and lengthen them. Foam rolling could be the answer. Try it and see whether it's easier to do the side step after rolling (see page 131).

# Side Plank and Mini Side Plank

This exercise is great for training your oblique abdominal muscles. By lying still, you make a very controlled movement and you can concentrate on your posture combined with your breathing. You slowly build it up from easy (whereby you use your oblique abdominal muscles for the first time again) to an extremely good exercise for those who are more advanced (to give you an amazing waistline).

**TAKE NOTE!**

- Place your elbow under your shoulder.
- Keep your butt forward: that's how you make a straight plank and not one with a kink.
- Keep your head in line with your spine.
- Keep your shoulders open.

## Levels:

1. The Mini Side Plank: Keep your knees on the floor. This is really helpful during the weeks after childbirth if you do not want to put too much pressure on the oblique abdominal muscles.
2. Support yourself with only your foot and lower arm.
3. Add a rotation.

# Side Slides ⓟ ⓓ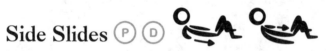

Time for those side abdominal muscles. This is a relatively easy exercise that gives you quick results. This is a real classic for good reason. It's also safe for your back because you decide whether to support it or not. When you stop using the floor for support, you also use your vertical abdominal muscles.

**TAKE NOTE!**

- Pay attention to your breathing and don't push. If you have a prolapse, pushing will only make it worse. If you can't keep breathing properly when doing this exercise, knock it down a level.
- Keep your back and shoulders parallel to the floor.
- When you think you have reached your maximum stretch point, stretch a little farther.
- Do not raise your head.

## Levels:

1. Keep your back on the floor.
2. With your shoulder blades off the floor.

# Sit-Ups Ⓟ Ⓓ ○←⅄ 

The basic of basic exercises for the abdominal muscles—this exercise trains your vertical abdominal muscles in particular. But don't be fooled: so many people don't do this so-called simple exercise properly . . . and then you are not really working out and you could damage your back or neck.

## Take note!
- Pull up using the strength of your abdominal muscles. Don't pull up with your neck, and make sure your back doesn't see-saw.
- Pay special attention to your breathing and do not push. Pushing is extremely bad, especially if you have a prolapse, because you put too much pressure on the pelvic floor.
- Roll up and roll down properly.

## Levels: Sit-Up +
1. Hands forward.
2. On shoulders.
3. Behind the ears.

**SELF-TEST & ACTIVATION:** If your body is preventing you from doing more or better Sit-Ups because you are finding it hard to roll up and down, then first use a foam roll to loosen your back (see page 131).

## Variation:
With a weight on your chest, or make it really challenging and hold the weight in front of your head.

# Split Squats (Lunges) Ⓟ

The names of these two exercises often get confused: Lunges and Split Squats. When you do this exercise standing still, it's called the Split Squats, when you walk (you shift your weight to the front leg in this position), then you are doing Lunges. Whatever they are called, they are tough going and real fat burners because they use such a large muscle group. You will also get a nice stretch at the front of your hips, which is often too short in many people. And as if that wasn't enough, it's also good for your stability.

## TAKE NOTE!
- Pay attention to your breathing and don't push to find your strength. Pushing is never good, especially if you have a prolapse!

- Keep your head in a neutral position; therefore, don't look at your toes.
- Keep your back in a neutral position and don't hollow it.
- Knees point to your toes and therefore not inward.
- Your feet point forward and are parallel.
- One knee under the hip and the other knee above the ankle.
- Drop the rear knee to the floor . . . and don't stop until you reach it.

## Levels: Split Squats +

1. Normal Split Squats.
2. On a raised surface with your front or back leg so that you can go deeper.
3. Now, add a jump!

## Variation:

With weights, jumping while alternating legs . . . there are endless variations.

**SELF-TEST & ACTIVATION:** Are you trying to go down as far as you can, but you automatically hollow your back and you can feel the top of your thigh pulling? If so, then try foam rolling the part that pulls. When it is relaxed and lengthened you will probably be able to do deeper Lunges in your neutral position. And the deeper you go, the more effective it is.

# Squat, Squat 'n' Walk, Mini Squat, Chair Squat Ⓟ

Squats really are the king of all exercises: they give you strong and nicely shaped legs, and you burn a massive number of calories because you are training such a large muscle group. Those well-trained leg muscles will help you lift your baby responsibly, also when baby is pounds heavier. You can start with Mini Squats early on. They are great in the first phase of recovery to start extending the leg muscles that often shorten during the pregnancy.

## TAKE NOTE!

- Pay attention to your breathing and don't push to get strength. Pushing is never good, especially if you have a prolapse!
- Keep your head in a neutral position; far too many people move their head backward when doing a Squat.
- Keep your back in a neutral position and don't roll down.

- Your knees should be facing your toes and not pointing inward or outward.

## Levels: Squat +

1. Don't go deeper than your knees.
2. Go as deep as possible.
3. Now, add a jump.

## Variations:

- With weights or an elastic band just above your knees.
- With a step in between: Squat 'n' Walk.

**SELF-TEST:** Your leg muscle may be restricted, preventing you from going as deeply as you would like. If so, try standing with your heels on something. A small height increase under your heels can work wonders. Try standing on a threshold when making a Squat. Does that help? If so, it means your calves are too short. From now on, you should foam roll them before doing Squats. Do the Squats with your heels on that threshold until you can do no more.

If you still can't manage the Squat properly, even on a threshold, then your hip may be stuck. Try and roll it loose. Loosening your hips can also help if your knees collapse inward (see page 131).

If it's not your calves stopping you from doing a good Squat but your knees fall inward, then activate your hips.

# Beginners Squat: Mini Squat ⓟ

You can do the Mini Squat instead of doing the Chair Squat. You do a Squat but not too deep. Go down a little and then back up again. Build it up slowly to a full Squat and take note: do not force anything during your recovery! It's better to do a good Mini Squat than a full Squat irresponsibly.

# Beginners Squat: Chair Squat ⓟ

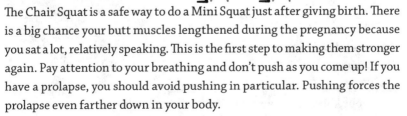

The Chair Squat is a safe way to do a Mini Squat just after giving birth. There is a big chance your butt muscles lengthened during the pregnancy because you sat a lot, relatively speaking. This is the first step to making them stronger again. Pay attention to your breathing and don't push as you come up! If you have a prolapse, you should avoid pushing in particular. Pushing forces the prolapse even farther down in your body.

## TAKE NOTE!
Use the strength from your legs and don't swing your body upward.

# Stretches

**NECK STRETCHES (HEAD TO SHOULDERS):** This is the way to relax your neck quickly. The weight of your hand on its own is enough.

**CALF STRETCHES:** Stretch your calves by standing on a threshold or slightly higher surface. It's great to do at any time. Our calves are often too short due to our lifestyle and wearing heels.

**CHEST AND SIDE BODY STRETCHES:** Stretch against a wall to keep from stretching too far, which would stretch your abdominal muscles too far and thereby further increase (any) diastasis. The flatter your hands are against the wall, the more you stretch.

**SHOULDER STRETCHES:** Make slow circles while standing tall so that you don't put extra pressure on your neck muscles.

# Sumo Squat ('n' Walk) ℗

As a variation of the Squat, this exercise does almost the same but with a slight difference. Because you stand with a twisted posture, you increase the flexibility in your hips. The Sumo Squat is a fat killer because you train the biggest muscle groups—your leg and butt muscles—with one exercise. And that's not the only benefit: it also gives you incredibly toned legs and buttocks. It's not an easy exercise, but it's a good one to get your heart rate up.

## TAKE NOTE!
- Pay attention to your breathing and don't push to gain strength that way. Pushing is never good, especially if you have a prolapse!
- Keep your head in a neutral position; far too many people move their head backward when doing a squat.
- Keep your neck in neutral position and don't roll down.
- Push your hips forward.
- Your knees face your toes, don't point them inward.

### Levels: Sumo Squat +

1. Don't go deeper than your knees.
2. Go as deep as possible.
3. Now, add a jump.

### Variations:

- With weights or an elastic band just above your knees.
- With a step in between: Sumo Squat 'n' Walk.

**SELF-TEST & ACTIVATION:** See Squat (page 286).

# Super Mom ⒟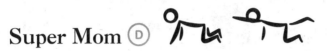

When your core stability meets your coordination with a touch of balance, then you are in Super Mom phase. It's so important to regain your balance after being out of balance with all those pregnancy pounds. This is a great exercise for that. Pay attention to keeping your torso still. It's difficult but great for regaining stability.

**TAKE NOTE!**

- Because this exercise starts from all fours you need to take care if you have a large diastasis. The pressure on the abdominal wall can get too much in this position. Stop if you feel any discomfort or pain.
- Don't hollow your back.
- Keep your head in a neutral position and don't look up!

# Table Top ⒟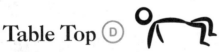

This exercise is helpful for anyone who sits at the computer a lot. It stretches the muscle groups that get stuck in a "computer posture" and you train the opposite muscle groups, which will give you a nice straight posture. And you will no longer be hindered by shortened muscles at the front of your body.

**TAKE NOTE!**

- If you have a large diastasis and feel discomfort or pain, then skip this exercise.
- Don't overstretch your elbows.
- Keep your back neutral and not hollow.
- Keep your head neutral; don't let it drop.

## Levels:

1. Normal Table Top.
2. Stretch one leg.
3. At its highest point, stretch your leg and hold it in position.

**SELF-TEST & ACTIVATION:**  If your abdominals have trouble holding the plank position while doing the Table Top, you would be better off activating your abdominal muscles first so that you will be able to do the exercise better and keep going for longer (see page 131).

# Triceps Dip ⓟ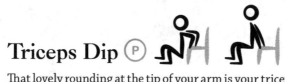

That lovely rounding at the tip of your arm is your triceps. There are numerous ways to train them, but dips are by far the easiest and best way because you can do them anywhere, even several times a day.

## TAKE NOTE!

- Move your back as close as possible to the object you are holding on to.
- Keep your back nice and neutral (straight).
- Keep your shoulders low and slightly back.
- Make sure your elbows don't move inward.

## Levels:

1. On something at hip height, such as a countertop.
2. On a chair.
3. With stretched legs.

# BEFORE AND AFTER

# BACK PHASE—WEEKS 0–6

Getting back to you starts with the "Back" phase. You take a little step back. Right now, it's about getting rest and making a connection: a connection with your baby and a connection with your new role as a mother. The exercises focus on the connection between your mind and your powerhouse.

## Fill the following in before the "Back" phase:

How fit do you feel?

☐ 1  ☐ 2  ☐ 3  ☐ 4  ☐ 5
☐ 6  ☐ 7  ☐ 8  ☐ 9  ☐ 10

How comfortable are you in your own skin?

☐ 1  ☐ 2  ☐ 3  ☐ 4  ☐ 5
☐ 6  ☐ 7  ☐ 8  ☐ 9  ☐ 10

Weight? _____

How many inches is your waistline? _____

Notes _____

# TO PHASE—WEEKS 7–24

In the "To" phase you gradually pick up your "normal" life again. You go back to work, to your social life, to yourself. The exercises work toward your stability and mobility.

## Fill the following in before the "To" phase:

How fit do you feel?

☐ 1  ☐ 2  ☐ 3  ☐ 4  ☐ 5
☐ 6  ☐ 7  ☐ 8  ☐ 9  ☐ 10

How comfortable are you in your own skin?

☐ 1  ☐ 2  ☐ 3  ☐ 4  ☐ 5
☐ 6  ☐ 7  ☐ 8  ☐ 9  ☐ 10

Weight? _____

How many inches is your waistline? _____

Notes _____

# YOU PHASE—WEEKS 25–39

You are increasingly becoming your "new you" and finding your own strength. The exercises work intensively on that new you so that you will be healthier, stronger (both mentally as well as physically), and in better shape. You will become your new "You!" Or perhaps even a better version of yourself than ever before.

### Fill the following in before the "You" phase:

How fit do you feel?

☐ 1 ☐ 2 ☐ 3 ☐ 4 ☐ 5
☐ 6 ☐ 7 ☐ 8 ☐ 9 ☐ 10

How comfortable are you in your own skin?

☐ 1 ☐ 2 ☐ 3 ☐ 4 ☐ 5
☐ 6 ☐ 7 ☐ 8 ☐ 9 ☐ 10

Weight?_____

How many inches is your waistline?_____

Notes_____

# BACK TO YOU—WEEK 40

No one can say exactly how long you will need to completely recover. One woman may be back to herself in nine months; another may need longer. But one thing is certain: since you have made it this far, you have been working extremely hard on yourself and you've earned these results.

### Fill the following in before Week 40:

How fit do you feel?

☐ 1 ☐ 2 ☐ 3 ☐ 4 ☐ 5
☐ 6 ☐ 7 ☐ 8 ☐ 9 ☐ 10

How comfortable are you in your own skin?

☐ 1 ☐ 2 ☐ 3 ☐ 4 ☐ 5
☐ 6 ☐ 7 ☐ 8 ☐ 9 ☐ 10

Weight?_____

How many inches is your waistline?_____

Notes_____

# AFTERWORD

It's done, you are . . . Back To You. You have gone through some journey and transition. We are honored to have been allowed to guide you on this journey. It's quite something. It was hard work and training, but you are now Back To You. Forty weeks ago, you made that first connection with your brain and pelvic floor muscles by visualizing them, and now you can jump on a trampoline with a full bladder. Reread your diary—you have accomplished something quite amazing! You should be proud of that. Immensely proud.

We hope that the BTY program has been a great help to you. We hope that your powerhouse has never been so powerful, that you have gained a habit for life in the BTY Kegel exercises, and that you have found your way in your body, mind, and motherhood.

Keep the XL Fundamentals as fundamental parts of your life. Keep paying attention to your nutrition, your posture, your breathing, your rest and relaxation, and never stop exercising and training.

Stay strong, stay healthy, stay . . . **YOU**.

With love,
XAVIERA AND LAURENS

# ACKNOWLEDGMENTS

An incredibly special thank you goes to all the global experts who have made it possible for us to compile this method. Without their expertise, and medical and often holistic viewpoints, we would never have been able to give this program the exceptional form it has.

*Dr. Sheila de Liz* (gynecologist, USA & Germany). Not only are you one of the leading experts, but you have also become a friend and my (Xaviera's) hero.

*Dr. Lindsey Vestal* (occupational therapist and pelvic floor expert, USA & France). Thank you for all your input, enthusiasm, and exceptional view of the pelvic floor and its relation to all other parts of the body. Our visit to Paris to see you not only enriched our book but also us as people.

*Dr. Sonia Bahlani* (gynecologist specializing in pelvic floor issues and urology, USA). Your holistic view of female health really opened our eyes. Your input has enabled this book to go to the next level.

*Dr. Miranda Goërtz* (psychologist, the Netherlands). Thanks for all your insights and support on all levels.

*Lars Mak* (singer and Estill Voice Trainer). Sound, vocalization, and posture: everything truly is connected.

*Ann-Marlene Henning* (sex and relationship therapist, Germany). What a wonderful, open, and down-to-earth view you have of sex and relationships. Every couple could learn something from that!

*Betül Berthold* (mental health coach, Germany). We had such an exciting discussion, and you have such good, specific ideas about how a woman can support herself.

*Patrick Johnson* (postural coordination expert, Alexander Technique, the Netherlands). What a refreshing and unique view you have of how behavior affects our posture!

*Nikki Ditrolio*, London's Pilates expert and queen of the "neutral spine."

*Caroline Poorterman* (midwife, the Netherlands). The world's best midwife and my dear friend.

*Dr. Judith Meer* (PT, DPT, PRPC, CSCS, pelvic floor therapist, USA). We still often think back to our meeting and the discussions in New York.

*Dr. Jolene Brighten* (naturopathic physician, biochemist, and expert in female hormones, USA). Jolene, there are few people who have the energy and fantastic gift to clarify the complex subject that every woman should know about. You are unique and a warrior for female awareness about everything in and around the body.

*Ralph Moorman* (engineer, nutritionist and food technologist, founder of the Hormone Factor Program, the Netherlands). You opened my (Laurens's) eyes when I made the connection between sport, diet, and hormones. I am proud to have you as my teacher.

*Kathelijne Mischner* (sports instructor, the Netherlands). Thanks, thanks, thanks. It was such a ball doing the recordings with you.

*Prof. Adriaan Honig* (psychiatrist, the Netherlands). An exceptional interview with an exceptional grandchild in his arms.

*Dr. Dorine van Ravensberg* (human movement scientist, the Netherlands). Thanks for you multiple rereads, your constructive criticism, and the insights you gave us.

*Dr. Frans Plooij.* My (Xaviera's) dearest father, adviser, support, and help. You are my hero.

It was an enormous and challenging puzzle, but after numerous discussions with scientists, experts, and physicians, we did it. You are holding the very first book that can genuinely help you recover from your amazing performance when you brought your little miracle into the world.

With love,
XAVIERA AND LAURENS

# BIBLIOGRAPHY

Bakken Sperstad, J., et al. "Diastasis Recti Abdominis during Pregnancy and 12 Months after Childbirth: Prevalence, Risk Factors and Report of Lumbopelvic Pain." *British Journal of Sports Medicine*, September 2016.

Abou-Saleh, M.T., et al. "Hormonal Aspects of Postpartum Depression." *Psychoneuroendocrinology*, July 1998.

American Psychological Association. "New Mothers Grow Bigger Brains within Months of Giving Birth: Warmer Feelings toward Babies Linked to Bigger Mid-brains." ScienceDaily, October 20, 2010.

Bancroft, J., et al. "The Dual Control Model: Current Status and Future Directions." *Journal of Sex Research* 46, nos. 2 and 3 (March–June 2009): 121–142.

Bastos, M. de, et al. "Combined Oral Contraceptives: Venous Thrombosis." *Cochrane Database of Systematic Reviews*, March 3, 2014.

Blackwell Publishing Ltd. "Women Report Sexual Problems A Full Year after Giving Birth; Health Problems Vary by Race." ScienceDaily, March 22, 2007.

Brubaker, L. "Postpartum Urinary Incontinence." *BMJ*, May 25, 2002.

Cohen, R., et al. "Twelve-Month Contraceptive Continuation and Repeat Pregnancy among Young Mothers Choosing Postdelivery Contraceptive Implants or Post Placental Intrauterine Devices." *Contraception*, February 2015.

Curtis K. M., et al. "U.S. Medical Eligibility Criteria for Contraceptive Use," *Recommendation Report*, July 2016.

Eason, E., et al. "Effects of Carrying a Pregnancy and of Method of Delivery on Urinary Incontinence: A Prospective Cohort Study." *BMC Pregnancy Childbirth*, February 19, 2004.

Fonti, Y., et al. "Postpartum Pelvic Floor Changes." *Journal of Prenatal Medicine*, October–December 2009.

"Giving Birth Changes a Mother's Brain. Here's How It Prepares Her for Raising Her Baby." *Business Insider*, 2019.

Glynn, L. M., and C. A. Sandman. "Prenatal Origins of Neurological Development: A Critical Period for Fetus and Mother." *Current Directions in Psychological Science*, December 5, 2011.

Hendrick, V., et al. "Hormonal Changes in the Postpartum and Implications for Postpartum Depression." *Psychosomatics*, March–April 1998.

Hoekzema, E., et al. "Pregnancy Leads to Long-Lasting Changes in Human Brain Structure." *Nature Neuroscience*, December 19, 2016.

Jackson E., et al. "Risk of Venous Thromboembolism during the Postpartum Period: A Systematic Review." *Obstetrics and Gynecology*, March 2011.

Johns Hopkins Medicine. "Delivery Method Associated with Pelvic Floor Disorders after Childbirth: Decade-Long Study Identifies Women at Highest Risk for Incontinence." ScienceDaily, December 19, 2018.

Kim, P. "Human Maternal Brain Plasticity: Adaptation to Parenting." *New Directions for Child and Adolescent Development*, September 2, 2016.

Loyola University Health System. "Majority of Women Report Sexual Dysfunction after Childbirth." ScienceDaily, November 26, 2014.

Madigan, D., and J. Shin. "Drospirenone-Containing Oral Contraceptives and Venous Thromboembolism: An Analysis of the FAERS Database." *Open Access Journal of Contraception*, April 2018.

Maintaining a Mindful Life (online course), Monash University, Australia.

McDonald, E. A., et al. "Dyspareunia and Childbirth: A Prospective Cohort Study." *BJOG: An International Journal of Obstetrics & Gynaecology*, April 2015.

McMaster University. "Urinary Incontinence Doubles Risk of Postpartum Depression." ScienceDaily, June 20, 2011.

*Medical Eligibility Criteria for Contraceptive Use*, 5th ed. (Geneva: World Health Organization, 2015).

Michigan Medicine, University of Michigan. "Half of Women over 50 Experience Incontinence, but Most Haven't Talked to a Doctor, Poll Finds: Urine Leakage Can Get in the Way of Life and Exercise; Results Point to Potential Importance of Routine Screening." ScienceDaily, November 1, 2018.

Muzik, M., et al. "PTSD Symptoms across Pregnancy and Early Postpartum among Women with Lifetime PTSD Diagnosis." *Depression and Anxiety*, July 2016.

Noonan, S., et al. "Food & Mood: A Review of Supplementary Prebiotic and Probiotic Interventions in the Treatment of Anxiety and Depression in Adults." *BMJ Nutrition, Prevention & Health*, July 6, 2020.

Ohio State University. "Immune System and Postpartum Depression Linked? Research in Rats Shows Inflammation in Brain Region after Stress during Pregnancy." ScienceDaily, November 6, 2018.

Ohio State University. "New Way to Think about Brain's Link to Postpartum Depression: Research in Animals Shows Brain's Immune System Is Activated by Stress during Pregnancy." ScienceDaily, October 21, 2019.

Parry, B. et al. "Sleep, Rhythms and Women's Mood. Part 1. Menstrual Cycle, Pregnancy and Postpartum." *Sleep Medicine Reviews*, April 2006.

"Pelvic Floor Dysfunction: Prevention and Non-surgical Management." Department of Health and Social Care in England, 2019.

"Rewiring the Brain for Happiness." Monash University, 2019.

Sacher, J., et al. "Elevated Brain Monoamine Oxidase A Binding in the Early Postpartum Period." *Archives of General Psychiatry*, May 2010.

Shlomi Polachek, I., et al. "Postpartum Post-Traumatic Stress Disorder Symptoms: The Uninvited Birth Companion." *IMAJ*, June 2012.

# Would You Like to Know More?

## More about your pelvic floor:

Dr. Lindsey Vestal, physiotherapist and pelvic floor specialist, United States and France

www.functionalpelvis.com

Kegels That Work: A Workshop for Women Who Want to Stop Guessing + Start Taking Back Control (https://ot-pioneers.teachable.com/p/kegelsthatwork)

Lindsey not only gives the best online lessons about your pelvic floor, but she also knows how to explain things in the nicest and best possible way.

## More about your body:

Dr. Sheila de Liz, gynecologist, United States and Germany

*Unverschämt, Alles über den fabelhaften weiblichen Körper* (Rowohlt Verlag, 2019)

www.dr-de-liz.de

*Woman on Fire: Alles über die fabelhaften Wechseljahre* (Rowohlt Verlag, 2020)

Sheila is a gynecologist who instantly becomes your friend. She is straight talking, whereby you suddenly understand your own body.

## More about relationships and sex:

Ann-Marlene Henning, sex and relationship therapist, Germany

www.doch-noch.de

*Sex verändert alles: Aufklärung für Fortgeschrittene* (Rowohlt Verlag, 2019)

*Wenn es um das Eine geht: Das Thema Sexualität in der Therapie* (Vandenhoeck & Ruprecht, 2018)

*Liebespraxis: Eine Sexologin erzählt* (Rowohlt 2017)

*Make More Love: Ein Aufklärungsbuch für Erwachsene* (Goldmann Verlag, 2018)

## More about hormones:

Dr. Jolene Brighten, naturopathic doctor, chemist, and expert in female hormones

www.drbrighten.com

*Beyond the Pill: A 30-Day Program to Balance Your Hormones, Reclaim Your Body, and Reverse the Dangerous Side Effects of the Birth Control Pill* (HarperOne, 2020)

Jolene makes indigestible information about hormones comprehensible and has the best and most informative hormone Instagram account in the world.

# INDEX

abdominal breathing
    diaphragm and pelvic floor, 23
    breathing properly and, 10
    Dorine van Ravensberg, 190
abdominal muscles
    Adductor Ball, 268
    Bicycle Crunches, 269
    Cat to Cow, 271
    Dead Bug, 272
    diastasis recti, 32–36
    diastasis recti, test concerning,
        262–63
    diastasis, types of, 263
    Double Crunches, 273
    Heel Drop, variation, 274
    hernias, 30
    Hyper Back (with twist), variation,
        275
    Inchworm, 276
    Leg Lift, 276
    linea alba and, 261
    Mountain Climbers, 277
    oblique, 24
    pelvis and, 22–25
    PF Lift 2, 279
    Plank, 279
    Side Plank and Mini Side Plank,
        284
    Side Slides, 284
    Sit-Ups, 285
    Stretches, 288
    transverse, 24
    vertical, 24
Adductor Ball, 268
adrenaline, 53–54
alcohol
    breastfeeding and, 161
    nutrition and, 75, 80
antibiotics, training and, 115
anxiety
    HADS test, 66
    postpartum anxiety, 67–68
    training and, 113
    walking, 110

baby holding, posture and, 102
back mobility, 265
back muscles, 25
    Cat to Cow, 265
    Curl Up and Down, 271
    downward dog, 206
    lifting and, 101
    mobility of, 265
    pelvis and, 22–23
    Plank, 279
    powerhouse, 22, 23, 25
    pregnancy and, 25
    stickers exercise, 166
    Wall Pull-Down, 280
    zipper exercise, 100
"Back" phase, 149
    Ann-Marlene Henning on, 156
    exercises and, 124, 139, 157–59
    relationship, 64
Bahlani, Sonia, 13
    cesarean section, 180
    frequent urination, 31
    vagina, pH level of, 43
Bancroft, John, 221
bathroom
    perfect visit to, 103
    position and, 103
    posture and, 96
    prolapse, 37
    pushing and, 38
Bear Crawl, 268
Berthold, Betül, "Back" tips, 155
Bicycle Crunches, 269
birth control shot, 173
blocks
    block 1, 158–64
    block 2, 164–69
    block 3, 182–87
    block 4, 188–93
    block 5, 194–99
    block 6, 200–5
    block 7, 206–11
    block 8, 212–17
    block 9, 224–29

blocks (*continued*)
  block 10, 230–35
  block 11, 236–41
  block 12, 242–47
  block 13, 248–53
blood loss, 151
blood pressure
  *Rhodiola rosea*, 55
  sex and, 50
  training and, 111, 113
Body Extension, 270
bones
  Espsom salts footbath, 251
  estradiol, 53
  posture and, 95
  training and, 111, 112
  walking, 110
booty weeks, 232
brain
  60 bpm, 184
  activating muscles and, 131
  birth trauma and, 177
  brain, hormone logic, 90
  breathing and, 166
  care and stress, 67
  chewing and, 197
  childbirth and, 12, 17, 61
  cortisol levels and, 55
  hormonal contraception, 173
  light and, 87
  mind, 19
  mom brain, 17–19
  nuts and, 79
  omega-3 and, 79
  pelvic floor and, 28, 137
  relaxation and, 90
  sex and, 50, 176
  stress and, 90
Brain–Pelvic Floor Connection (lying down), 270
Brain–Pelvic Floor Connection (on hands and knees), 270
bread, 85, 239
breast milk
  alcohol, 161
  cabbage, 79
  caffeine, 161
  "honest" products, 75
  oligosaccharides, 85

orgasm, 46
oxytocin, 53
thyroid gland, 59
breastfeeding
  cabbage, 78
  cycle and, 175
  D-mannose, 80
  dieting, 219–20
  drinking water and, 155, 185
  engorgement, 150
  IUD, 174
  nutrition and, 161
  oxytocin, 53
  painful breasts, 150
  periods and, 56
  posture and, 100
  prolactin, 54, 56
  stretching during, 244
  uterine cramps, 150
  uterus, 156
  weight and, 57–58
breasts, 46
  engorgement, 150
  orgasm, 46
  posture and, 100
  uterus and, 156
breathing, 104–7
  abdominal breathing, 106
  body strain and, 105
  BTY Kegel exercises and, 139
  chest breathing, 106
  deacidification, 105
  detoxing and, 105
  diaphragm, 23–24
  digestion and, 105
  dildo and, 138
  dry mouth and, 117
  empty belly, 106
  energy and, 105
  exercise and, 109, 115, 226
  heart, 106
  hormones and, 105
  lifting and, 101
  lymphatic system, 105
  meditation, 167, 178
  midriff and, 184
  mouth breathing, 107
  nasal breathing, 107
  neck and head issues, 105

paraspinal muscles, 100
pelvic floor and, 166, 279
posture and, 94–95, 166, 196
pregnancy and, 101
proper breathing, 106
relaxing and, 155
stickers and, 166
stress and, 105, 155
3D breathing, 190
towel and, 190
XL breathing, 106–7, 190
Brighten Jolene
  cabbage, 79
  cortisol, 55
  food sensitives, 77
  gut microbiome, 81
  light, 88
  sex, 50
  "To" phase, 173
"Bring Sally Up, Bring Sally Down," 238
BTY Kegel exercises, 139–44
  "Back" phase, 157
  calendar, 124
  golden rules for, 142
  pelvic floor, 121, 141
  powerhouse, 137
  "To" phase, 181
  trigger points, 143–44
  variations of, 142
  "You" phase, 223
BTY program
  basic principles of, 15
  connections, 13
  first phase, "Back," 149–69
  insight and reassurance, 14
  second phase, "To," 171–217
  third phase, "You," 219–57
  three phases of, 14
  XL impact, 13
B vitamins, 80, 84

cabbage, 78, 79, 84, 150
calves, 99, 208, 287, 288
care, stress and, 67
caregiver, 171
casein, 77
Cat to Cow, 265–66, 271
cervical cap, 38
cesarean section, 179

bladder, 180
  exercises and, 124
  pelvic floor muscles, 26
  recovering from, 152
  uterine cramps, 150
  vagina and, 41, 44
  vertical abdominal muscles, 134
Chair Squat, 286
changes
  doubting yourself more than ever, 65
  forgetting your relationship, 64
  forgetting yourself, 62
  increased sensitivity, 61
  new job?, 62–64
  reconsidering norms and values, 62
  setting the bar too high, 65
  social network, 64
chest breathing, 106, 184
clitoris
  blood flow, 44–45
  clitoral orgasm, 48–49
  prolapse, 37, 175
coffee, 75, 80, 146, 161
cold showers, 214
condoms, 44, 174
contraception, after childbirth, 172–73
contraction, 53, 150
cortisol, 53–55
  kissing, 250
  sex and, 50
  stress, 57
  training and, 114
crying
  baby blues, 70, 151
  crying/baby blues, 151
  postpartum depression and, 69–70,
    151
"cuddle hormone," 53
cup of coffee, 146, 161
Curl Up and Down, 271

day-night rhythm, sleep and, 87
deacidification, breathing and, 105
Dead Bug, 272
demanding functionality, 128, 130, 134
depression, 65–70
  Honig, Adriaan, 66
  hormonal contraception, 173
  thyroid gland, 58

depression (*continued*)
training and, 113
walking, 110
*See also* postpartum depression, 69
detoxing, breathing and, 105
diaphragm (cervical cap), 38
diaphragm (midriff), 22–24
abdominal breathing and, 106
breathing practices, 24
during pregnancy, 106
pelvic floor and, 22
posture and, 99
powerhouse and, 22–23, 107
stress and, 24
XL breathing, 106–7
diary
block 1, 162–63
block 2, 168–69
block 3, 186–87
block 4, 192–93
block 5, 198–99
bock 6, 204–5
block 7, 210–11
bock 8, 216–17
block 9, 228–29
block 10, 234–35
block 11, 240–41
block 12, 246–47
block 13, 252–53
week 40, 256–57
diastasis, muscles
back phase exercises and, 124
linea alba and, 32
positions of, 33
posture and, 94–95
powerhouse and, 22, 30, 32
preganancy, effects on, 32
stretching and, 134
switchblade motion and, 98
testing of, 261
"To" phase training and, 180
types of, 263
diastasis recti, 32
developing, chance of, 33
linea alba and, 32
types of, 33
dieting, 219–22
digestion
breathing and, 105
chewing and, 197

mint tea and, 209
diindolylmethane (DIM), 78
dildo
G-spot, 49
pelvic floor muscles and, 138
vagina, confidence in, 45–46
DIM, 78
disorders, psyche and, 67
D-mannose, 80
domino effect, 39
dopamine
sex and, 50
training and, 114
Double Crunches, 273
"doubteritis," 17
Downward Dog, 272
dry brushing, 208
dual control model, 47, 221

earlobes, 238
edema, 98
endorphins, 53
energy
breastfeeding and, 161
breathing and, 105
cold showers and, 214
dry brushing, 208
earlobes and, 238
eating schedule and, 167
nutrition, the mind and, 155
posture and, 95
stress and, 105
sugar and, 76
testosterone and, 54
training and, 112
engorgement, 150–51
episiotomy, 152
Epsom salts, 251
erogenous zone, earlobes, 238
estradiol, 53
estriol, 43, 53, 175
Estriol cream, 43, 175
estrogen, 53
ailments and, 56
cabbage, 78
estrogen-like substances, 82
gut microbiome and, 81
stress and, 57
weight and, 57–58
estrone, 53

exercising, 109–111
  back exercises, 100
  "Back" exercises, 119
  breathing and, 115
  diastasis recti, 35
  exercise standard, 109
  healthcare provider and, 11
  posture and 95
  prolapse, 38
  "To" exercises, 119
  training and, 111, 115
  walking, 110
  XL Fundamentals and, 72
  "You" exercises, 119
  See also BTY Kegel exercises and
    training

facial yoga, 191
FAM, 174
feet
  bootbath, 251
  edema, 98
  muscles in, training of, 214
  position of, pelvic floor and, 99, 202
  posture and 94
fermentation, 78, 84
fertility awareness method (FAM), 174
fiber-rich foods, 75, 79, 150
finger gymnastics, 250
first training session, 119–22
flaxseed, 232–33
  omega-3, 79
  salads and, 239
  smoothies and,, 227
food, 75–85
  avoiding meat, 215
  breastfeeding and, 161, 220
  chewing, 197
  constipation, 150
  dieting, 219–22
  eating mindfully, 202–3
  estrogens, 82
  gut microbiome and, 81
  healthcare provider, 11
  healthy, 155
  iron, 191
  monosodium glutamate, 83
  nutrition tips, 75
  plasticizers, 82
  prebiotics, 85

protein, 191
rainbow, 245
reset days and, 92
spread food out, 167
footbath, 251
fructo-oligosaccharides (FOS), 85

galacto-oligosaccharides (GOS), 85
gluten, 77
Goërtz, Miranda
  mother-baby connection, 154
  re-birthing, 176–77
  yourself and your strength, 222
gravity
  diastasis recti, 35
  standing and, 98
  training and, 116
G-spot, 48–49
gut flora
  brain and, 81
  B12 deficiency and, 80
  fiber-rich foods, 79
  pickles and, 84
gut microbiome
  brain and, 81
  B12 and, 80
  prebiotics and, 79, 85
  probiotics and, 84

HADS test, 66
hair loss, 151
happiness, 90–91, 196
heart
  cold water and, 214
  omega-3, 232
  pregnancy and, 106
  stairs, 226
  thyroid gland, 58
  walking, 110
heartburn, 250
Heel Drop, 273
Heel Slide, 274
hemorrhoids, 103, 150
Henning, Ann-Marlene
  "Back" tips, 156
  dual control model, 47
  "To" phase, 175
  "You" tips, 221
hernia, 22, 30–32, 39, 94
hernia umbilicus, 30

high-intensity interval training (HIIT), 54
Hip Abductor, 274
hippocampus, 90
Hoekzema, Elseline, 18
Holmes, Thomas, 67
Holmes and Rahe, 259
"honest" products, 75
Honig, Adriaan, depression, 66
hormonal contraception, 173
hormones, 52–59
    adrenaline, 53–54
    baby blues, 151
    brain and, 18
    breathing and, 105
    cortisol, 53–55, 57
    diastasis, 32
    estrogen, 53, 56
    human growth hormone, 54
    incontinence, 52
    meditation, 166
    new levels of, 12
    oxytocin, 53
    postpartum depression, 52
    postpartum thyroiditis, 58
    production of, 56
    progesterone, 151
    prolactin, 54
    regaining balance of, 57
    relaxin, 55
    sleep, 87, 90
    stress, 77, 87, 105
    testosterone, 54
    training and, 111, 113–14
    walking, 110
    water, 155
    what are they, 52
    why learn about, 52
    Xenoestrogens, 82
    XL Fundamentals and, 126
human growth hormone (HGH), 54, 87
Hyper Back (with twist), 275

Ice Skaters, 275
immune system
    antibiotics, 115
    baby's, 75
    cabbage, 78
    cold water, 214
    food and, 77
    gut microbiome, 81
    sex and, 50
    vitamin C-1000, 80
imprint position, 147
Inchworm, 276
incisions, 152
incontinence
    gut microbiome and, 81
    hormones and, 52
    pelvic floor muscles and, 12, 29
    scar tissue, 180
intrauterine device (IUD), 173
inulin, 85
IUD, 173

Janssen, Erick, 221
Johnson, Patrick, posture, 104
juices, 227

kefir, 84
Kegel, Arnold, 139
Kegel exercises, 139–44
kimchi, 78
kissing, 250

lacerations, 152
lactose, 77, 84
Leg Lift, 276
lemon water, 250
levator ani, 203
lifting
    alternating left and right, 160
    posture and, 101, 146
linea alba, 32–34, 261–62
Liz, Sheila de
    "Back" tips, 154
    prolapse, 37
    superstrength, 63
    "To" phase, 174–75
    "You" tips, 221
loose neck, 96
losing fluids, 151
lymphatic system, 105
    exercise and, 139, 244
    lemon water, 250
    pelvic floor and, 179

magnesium
  knots and, 31
  muscle relaxation and, 29
  pelvic floor muscles, 80
  sunflower seeds, 79
Marconi Union, 184
meat
  avoidance of, 215
  protein and, 191
  substitutes, 83
  sugar and, 76
medication, 80, 126
meditation, 166–67, 177
  Berthold Betül, 155
  Miranda Goërtz, 177
  sleep and, 90
Meer, Judith, 36
melatonin
  light and, 88, 89
  sleep and, 55, 89–90
menstrual cycle
  insulin, 77
  light, 88
  pregnancy, 172
  sleep, 88
metabolism, training, 112
midriff (diaphragm)
  diastasis recti, 34
  loosening, 184
  posture, 99
  powerhouse, 22–24
milk substitutes, 83
mini pill, 173
Mini Squat, 286
mirror, 166
miso, 84
mom brain, 17–19
monosodium glutamate, 83
Mountain Climbers, 277
mouth breathing, 107
muscles
  activating, how to, 131–32
  activating, loosening, and demanding functionality, 128–35
  cesarean section, 134
  demanding functionality, 130, 134
  diastasis, 134
  knots, 133

  loosening, how to do it, 131–33
  "memory" of, 130
  muscles knots, 133
  pelvic, recovery of, 12
  relaxation of, magnesium, 29
  restricted muscle function, 128
  stretching and, 131, 133
  training and, 111, 112
myofascial release, 36

Namaste, 277
NASA, 88
nasal breathing, 107
navel hernias, 30
neck, 96, 104, 105, 135
night sweats, 151
nutrition, 75–85
  alcohol, 80
  bread, 239
  breastfeeding and your food, 161
  cabbage, 78
  carbohydrates, refined, 76
  chewing, 197
  coffee, 80
  eating schedule, 167
  fiber-rich foods, 79
  flaxseed, 232
  fluids, 185
  fructo-oligosaccharides, 85
  galacto-oligosaccharides, 85
  "honest" products, 75
  inulin, 85
  iron, 191
  juices, 227
  kefir, 84
  lemon water, 250
  meat, 215
  milk, 83
  mindful eating, 202
  miso, 84
  monosodium glutamate, 83
  nonprescription medication, 80
  nutritional supplements, 80
  nuts, 79
  organic food, 76
  pectin, 85
  pickles, 84
  postpartum depression, 13, 70

nutrition (*continued*)
  probiotics, 84
  protein, 191
  sauerkraut, 84
  seeds, 79
  smoking, 80
  smoothies, 227
  soy, 83
  sugar, 76
  tea, 209
  10 golden tips, 75
  vegetables, 78
  yogurt, 84
nuts, 79
  amino acids, 191
  GOS, 85

omega-3, 79, 232–33
organic food, 76
orgasm
  breasts and, 46
  definition of, 49
  drugs, effects on, 43
  four types of, 48
  pelvic floor muscles, 12, 29, 44
  prolactin, 50
oxygen
  energy, 105
  optimum levels of, 94
  posture and, 94–95
oxytocin, 53
  breastmilk, 46
  kissing, 250
  sex and, 45
  uterine cramps, 150

painful breasts (engorgement), 150
pectin, 85
Pelvic Bridge, 278
pelvic floor exercises
  extra, dynamic, 227
  extra, jumping, 238
  extra, tightening and relaxing, 209
  orgasms and, 49
  pain and, 143
pelvic floor muscles, 26
  brain and, 28
  breathing exercises and, 28
  detailed view of, 27
  diastasis recti, 32–36
  embarrassment and pleasure, 26
  exercises, 137–44
  feet and, 99
  frequent urination, 31
  knots, 143–44
  location, 137
  main functions of, 26
  orgasm, 44
  pressure during pregnancy, 30–39
  pregnancy and, 26–27
  prolapse, 36–39
  sore pelvic floor, 150
  tensing of, 142
  test of all tests, 257
  tightening and relaxing, 28–29
  trigger points, 143–44
pelvis. *See* pelvic floor muscles
perfection, 91
PF Lift 1, 278
PF Lift 2, 279
phytoestrogens, 82
pickles, 84
pill, the, 173
Plank, 279
post-traumatic stress disorder (PTSD),
  68
postpartum anxiety, 68, 110
postpartum contractions, 53, 150
postpartum depression, 69–70
  birth control shot, 173
  gut microbiome, 81
  hormones, 52
  incontinence and, 29
  nutrition and, 13
  walking, 110
postpartum health issues, 150
postpartum psychosis, 69
postpartum stress, 67
postpartum thyroiditis, 58
posture, 94–103
  abdominal cavity, 32
  appearance and, 95
  bathroom trips and, 96
  Body Extension, 270
  bones and, 95
  calf time, 208
  carrying your child, 101
  Cat to Cow, 265

diastasis, 32, 34
Downward Dog, 272
feet and, 99
holding your baby, 102
imitate your baby, 196
imprint position, 146–47
lifting and, 101
loose neck, 96
mirror exercise, 166
muscle strain and, 95
neck and, 96
neutral position, 146–47
oxygen and, 94
Patrick Johnson, 104
Plank, 279
powerful appearance and, 95
powerhouse and, 95
pregnancy posture, 25
prolapse, 37
Reverse Fly (sitting or standing), 281
Row, 282
shoes, 202
sitting and, 37, 97–98
sore pelvic floor, 150
standing, 37, 98–99
Table Top, 289
tips for, 100
toe gymnastics, 214
toilet position, 37, 103
training and, 111, 113, 116, 146–47
training method, correct, 95
Wall Pull-Down, 280
zipper exercise, 100
power naps, sleep and, 88
powerhouse, 22–25
  Adductor Ball, 268
  breathing and, 106–7
  Cat to Cow, 271
  Dead Bug, 272
  diastasis and, 32
  domino effect, 39
  lifting and, 101–2
  Namaste, 277
  posture and, 94
  pressure and, 30, 38
  prolapse and, 36
  proper use of, 95
  Wall Pull-Down, 280
prebiotics, 79, 84, 85

pressure distribution, 38, 120
probiotics, 78, 84
progesterone
  baby blues, 151
  IUDs and, 173
  pregnancy and, 56
  relaxin and, 55
  stress, 57
  testosterone, 54
progestin, 173
progestogen-only pill (mini pill), 173
prolactin, 50, 54, 56
prolapse (sagging), 36–39, 175
  baby lifting and, 101
  PF Lift 1, 278
  PF Lift 2, 279
  powerhouse and, 30, 95
  test, 264
psyche, disorders and, 67
PTSD, 68–69
Push-Ups, 280

Rahe, Richard, 67
Ravensberg, Dorine van, breathing, 190
relationship, 47, 64, 70, 174, 221
relaxation, 90–92
  facial yoga, 191
  lavender, 177
  mom's mini meditation, 166
  pitfalls to, 91
  relaxin, 55
  screen downtime, 226
  total relaxation, 160
  "Weightless," 184
relaxin, 55
reset day, 92
Reverse Fly (sitting or standing), 281
*Rhodiola rosea* (rose root), 55
rose root, 55
Round the Clock Lunges, 282
Row, 282

sagging. *See* prolapse
Salamander, 283
sauerkraut, 84
scars, 42–43, 178, 180
screen downtime, 226
screens, sleep and, 88
seeds, 79, 191, 233

serotonin, 50, 90, 110
sex, 42
  benefits for women, 50
  desire, lack of, 46
  mood change, 48
  oxytocin, 53
  relationship, change in, 47
shoes, 202, 214
Side Lunges, 283
Side Plank and Mini Side Plank, 284
Side Slides, 284
sitting, 97
Sit-Ups, 285
skin
  chemicals on, 82
  Epsom salts, 251
  training and, 111, 114
sleep, 87–90
  baby sleep, 155
  day-night rhythm, 87
  difficulty with, 244
  hormones, 13
  magnesium, 29
  power naps, 88–89
  screens and, 88
smoking, 75, 80
smoothies, 78, 227, 233
social life, 92, 119, 232
sore pelvic floor, 150
soy, 82–84
Split Squats (lunges), 285
spontaneity, 91
sports, 208
sports club, 208
Squat, 286
Squat 'n' Walk, 286
squats, 286–87
stability
  pelvic floor muscle, 29
  stability training, 239
  transverse abdominal muscle and,
    24
stairs, 226
standing, 98–99
  booty weeks, 232
  mirror exercise, 166
  neck while, 96
  posture while, 37

Reverse Fly (sitting or standing),
  281
spine during, 147
Split Squats, 285
Stretches, 288
stretching, 244
stickers, 166
stress, 65–70
  breathing and, 105, 155
  care and, 67
  cortisol, 53, 114
  dehydration, 55
  diaphragm, 24
  earlobe, 238
  Epsom salts footbath, 251
  hormones, 53, 57
  kissing, 250
  meditation, 166, 177
  oxytocin, 250
  post-traumatic stress disorder
    (PTSD), 68
  postpartum anxiety, 68
  postpartum depression, 69–70
  postpartum psychosis, 69
  postpartum stress, 67
  psyche, 67
  sex, 50
  tea, 209
  test, 259
Stretches, 288
stretching, 244
sugar, 76–77
Sumo Squat ('n' Walk), 288
sunbathing, 202
super mom, 289
switchblade, 98

Table Top, 289
tampons, 82
tea, 209
tear, 152
ten-second time-out, 214–15
test
  breathing, 264–65
  diastasis recti, 261–63
  linea alba, 261–63
  pelvic floor muscles, 260
  prolapse, 264

stressful life events, 259
testosterone, 54, 114
three Cs, 17–19
thumbs, 102, 160
thyroid gland, 58–59, 70
time-out, 214–15
toe gymnastics, 214
toilet position, 96, 103
"To" phase
  Ann-Marlene Henning, 175
  BTY Kegel exercises, 181
  rebirthing, 177
  relationship and, 64
  training in, 180
tracking method (fertility awareness
  method), 174
training, 111–17
  antibiotics and, 115
  "Back" phase, 157
  basic posture, 146–47
  blood pressure, 113
  bones, 112
  breathing and, 115
  correct method of, 95
  dopamine and, 114
  exercise, 111
  fitness levels, 113
  metabolism, 112
  muscles and, 112
  skin and, 114
  10 golden tips, 115–16
  testosterone and, 114
  "To" phase, 180
  "You" phase, 222–23
transverse abdominal muscles, 24
  Adductor Ball, 268
  diastasis recti, 34
  Heel Drop, 273–74
  Leg Lift, 276
  Plank, 279
Triceps Dip, 290
trigger points, 31, 143–44
20/20/20 eye rule, 226

unintentional "foods," 80
urination
  disrupted urination reflex, 138
  frequent, 31

losing fluids, 151
pelvic floor muscles, 137
tears or incisions, 152
uterine cramps (postpartum contractions), 150
uterus, 25, 53, 156

vagina, 41–50
  birthing, recovery, 41
  "blocking", 264
  blood flow, 44–45
  BTY Kegel exercises and, 142
  confidence in, 45
  extra pelvic floor tip, 215
  feeling, reduced or lack, 261, 264
  "full" feeling, 264
  moisture, 29, 175
  noise, 264
  oat bath, 184
  orgasm, 48–49
  pain, 260
  pelvic floor and, 27, 31, 137–38
  penetration, 45–46
  pH level, 43–44
  prolapse, 37
  protrusion, at opening of, 260
  scars, 42–43, 178–79
  sensitivity, 44
  sore pelvic floor, 150
  tampons and, 264
  tear, recovering from, 152
  traumas and emotions, 47
  trigger points, 31, 143–44
  urination, 31
  vaginal dilator, 46
  vaginal orgasm, 48
"vaginal wind," 44
vegetables
  amino acids and, 191
  daily amount of, 78, 215
  fiber and, 79–80
  iron, 191
  juices, 227
  nutrition tips, 78
  prebiotics and, 85
  protein, 191
  rainbow, 245
  smoothies, 227

Vestal, Lindsey, 143, 178, 190
vitamin C
  immune system, 80
  iron, 191
  lemon water, 250
  sauerkraut, 84
vitamin D
  sunbathing, 202
  sunlight, 90
  vagina, 43
  walking, 110
vitamin E, 79, 178

walking, 110
  BTY Kegel exercises and, 142
  domino effect and, 39
  exercise, block 5, 196
  mirror exercise, 166
  pelvic floor exercises and, 224, 227
  posture and, 95–96
  vitamin D and, 202
  walking, shoes and, 202
Wall Pull-Down, 280
week 40, 223, 254–57
weight, 219–22
  baby holding, 102
  breathing and, 105
  cold water, 214
  Epsom salt footbath, 251
  estrogen and, 57
  high fructose syrup, 77
  human growth hormone (HGH) and, 54
  losing, 219–20
  pelvic floor muscles and 27
  posture and, 100
  sitting and, 97
  thyroid gland and, 58–59
  training, 111, 112
"Weightless," 184

work
  back to, 171–72
  career choices, 62–64, 259

Xenoestrogens, 82
XL Breath, 106–7
  brain pelvic floor connection and, 28
  BTY Kegel exercises and, 139, 141
  BTY workout and, 120
  midriff and, 184
  pregnancy and, 101
  XL breathing, 106
XL fundamentals, 13, 72–73, 124
  block 1, 160–61
  block 2, 166–67
  block 3, 184–85
  block 4, 190–91
  block 5, 196–97
  block 6, 202–3
  block 7, 208–9
  block 8, 214–15
  block 9, 226–27
  block 10, 232–33
  block 11, 238–39
  block 12, 244
  block 13, 250–51
  BTY workout and, 120
  exercise and training, 109–17
  nutrition, 75–85
  posture and breathing, 94–107
  rest and relaxation, 86–92
  variations for full control, 142
XL motion, 116, 120, 128

yogurt, 84
"You" phase
  connection exercises, 139
  Miranda Goërtz, 222
  training in, 222–23